NEW DIRECTIONS FOR MENTAL HEALTH SERVICES

Inpatient Psychiatry in the 1990s

John P. Docherty
University of California, Los Angeles

EDITOR

Number 63, Fall 1994

JOSSEY-BASS PUBLISHERS
San Francisco

INPATIENT PSYCHIATRY IN THE 1990S
John P. Docherty (ed.)
New Directions for Mental Health Services, no. 63
H. Richard Lamb, Editor-in-Chief

Microfilm copies of issues and articles are available in 16mm and 35mm, as well as microfiche in 105mm, through University Microfilms Inc., 300 North Zeeb Road, Ann Arbor, Michigan 48106-1346.

LC 87-646993 ISSN 0193-9416 ISBN 0-7879-9990-3

NEW DIRECTIONS FOR MENTAL HEALTH SERVICES is part of The Jossey-Bass Social and Behavioral Science Series and is published quarterly by Jossey-Bass Inc., Publishers, 350 Sansome Street, San Francisco, California 94104-1342.

EDITORIAL CORRESPONDENCE should be sent to the Editor-in-Chief, H. Richard Lamb, Department of Psychiatry and the Behavioral Sciences, U.S.C. School of Medicine, 1934 Hospital Place, Los Angeles, California 90033-1071.

Cover photograph by Wernher Krutein/PHOTOVAULT © 1990.

Manufactured in the United States of America. Nearly all Jossey-Bass books, jackets, and periodicals are printed on recycled paper that contains at least 50 percent recycled waste, including 10 percent postconsumer waste. Many of our materials are also printed with vegetable-based inks; during the printing process, these inks emit fewer volatile organic compounds (VOCs) than petroleum-based inks. VOCs contribute to the formation of smog.

Contents

Editor's Notes

This volume is about practical issues in contemporary inpatient psychiatry. In recent years, inpatient care has undergone enormous change, and it will continue to undergo change for the immediate future, change which is bringing great strain. There have been financial pressures and increased clinical pressures in terms of the acuity of the patients being seen, more restricted time frames within which care must be provided, limitations in staff, and the necessity to develop and learn innovative ways to deliver care to very ill patients more efficiently. This volume focuses on some of the essential aspects of care in this new environment.

Chapter One reviews the two-hundred-year history of inpatient psychiatry in the United States and places contemporary changes in their intellectual, historic, and political context. The purpose of this chapter is to help those who are currently managing or working in inpatient psychiatry today to understand the historical forces and social and political processes that have led to the current state of affairs, to have a clear focus of the current tasks of inpatient psychiatry, and to lay a broad foundation for planning and participating in the future of this work. Chapter One also outlines the essential current tasks, clinical and administrative, that must be addressed by inpatient programs if they are to adapt to and help forward future mental health care in the United States.

Chapter Two discusses the evolution and expansion of managed care as an important regulatory structure for inpatient psychiatry. Specifically, this chapter discusses the forces that led to the emergence of managed care, the developmental process of the managed care entities, and their focus on improving the value of mental health care services. Chapter Three then describes some of the core clinical functions of an inpatient psychiatric facility operating in this managed care era. Specific attention is given to the function for which inpatient psychiatry has demonstrated efficacy, namely, short-term symptom suppression. Additionally, the importance of rapid and precise diagnosis, psychoeducation, family involvement, and posthospital planning is discussed.

Chapters Four through Six focus on the treatment of important specific clinical populations that are likely to be seen in the inpatient setting. Chapter Four reviews the scope of the problem of dual diagnosis, the relationships between psychiatric disorders and chemical dependence, brief assessment and intervention approaches for dual diagnosis psychiatric inpatients, and relapse prevention methods. Chapter Five discusses the comorbid medical problems with which psychiatric patients frequently present and describes recommended diagnostic and treatment regimens for some of the more common illnesses. Chapter Six concludes this section with a discussion of the management of disruptive patients. The difficulties commonly encountered on an inpatient psychiatric unit due to disruptive or otherwise difficult patients are described in the context of borderline personality disorder. Promising therapeutic techniques and staff education strategies are also presented.

The final section, Chapters Seven and Eight, focuses on some non-clinical activities that are conducted in an inpatient psychiatric facility. Chapter Seven discusses the importance of value, quality accounting, and outcomes management in the current era of care. Measurement tools and techniques are discussed in detail. Chapter Nine concludes the volume with a discussion of critical legal issues currently affecting inpatient psychiatric facilities and their effective management. Specific emphasis is placed on the importance of the informed consent process as a way to both facilitate treatment and prevent adverse legal outcomes.

John P. Docherty
Editor

JOHN P. DOCHERTY, M.D., is professor of clinical psychiatry and medical director of the Mental Health Group at the University of California, Los Angeles.

PART ONE

The Evolution of Inpatient Psychiatry

The history of the remarkable changes inpatient psychiatry has undergone during the past 200 years reveals repeated cyclical efforts to reduce cost, improve quality, and increase access; yet a myriad of problems remain that must be addressed if we are to more realistically and successfully plan the future of inpatient care.

Two Hundred Years of Inpatient Psychiatry

John P. Docherty

We are now at a culmination point in the 200-year history of the evolution of institutional psychiatry in the United States. This chapter will review that history and its implications for the current functions and form of inpatient psychiatry in the United States and will delineate the key functions that inpatient psychiatry must address in order to successfully adapt to the current era.

The history of U.S. hospital psychiatry is an interesting and, in many ways, remarkably orderly one. It has been marked by two very clear processes: first, progressive concern about cost and consequent underfunding of the service structure, leading to substantial and progressively intolerable human abuses, evidenced by poor quality services and/or inadequate access to services, and rectified by a process of cost shifting (particularly of the costs associated with the chronic and indigent patient); and second, the influence of new knowledge on the development of new treatment structures, which by and large disaggregated the unity and location of services originally assigned to hospital care. Figure 1.1 is a schematic diagram of the unfolding of this history.

Phase One, 1790–1840: The Asylum and the Introduction of Inpatient Psychiatry

Formal care for mental patients in the United States began with the introduction of philanthropic asylums. These institutions were derived from the seminal work in the 1790s of Philippe Pinel, a French psychiatrist, and William Tuke, a British reformer. Both conceived of an institution, a "retreat" as Tuke called it, that would provide for the dual functions of refuge and recuperation. The basic concept entailed providing a safe, caring, orderly, and quiet physi-

Figure 1.1. History of Inpatient Psychiatry

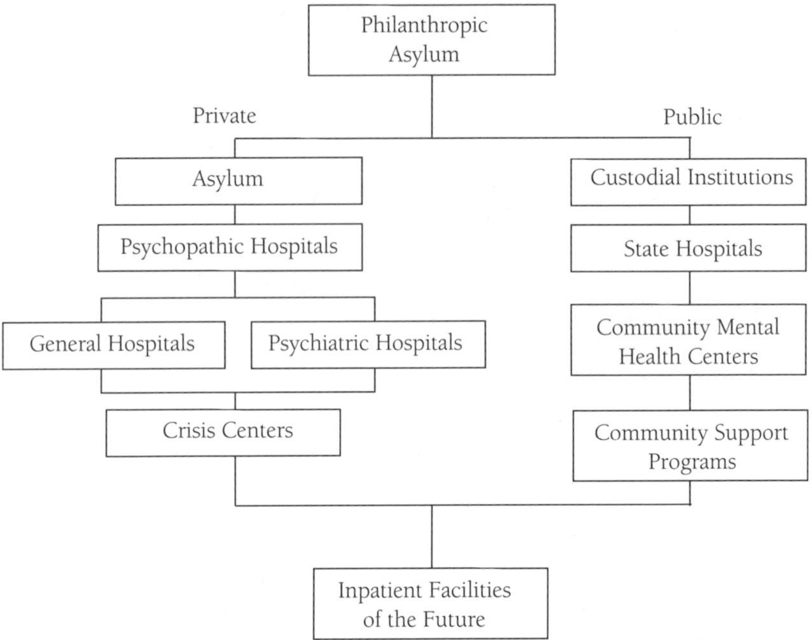

cal and social environment in which relationships of concern and wise guidance could be developed. The Pennsylvania Hospital, established in 1751, took on this cast. Beginning in 1813, a series of institutions were established along a similar model, including Friends Hospital in Pennsylvania, McLean Hospital in Massachusetts, and Bloomingdale in New York, followed by the Hartford Retreat, established in Connecticut in 1824. In general, these institutions were quite successful, with most patients discharged as "recovered" after a hospitalization of approximately three to nine months. Less than 15 percent of their populations were "custodial" patients (Grob, 1992).

At these asylums, individuals were provided the full range of care: they could be admitted for crisis, for a period of treatment and recuperation, or for treatment and recuperation followed by a more extended stay to facilitate the development of sufficient skills necessary to function successfully upon return to the community. Also, for those individuals who were unable to recover, an environment of protection and support was provided. Under this system, the functions of crisis stabilization, treatment, rehabilitation, and sanctuary were provided by one entity, in one location.

The success of these institutions, however, threatened to be overwhelmed by the progressive waves of immigration beginning in the 1840s. The indigency rates of the new populations as well as their sheer numbers threatened to overcome the philanthropically supported asylums. Such institutions, in order to maintain their character, needed to set limits on the numbers and types of patients they accepted. Therefore, new institutions needed to be developed to care for these now large numbers of indigent mentally ill individuals.

The drive to build such new institutions, which could provide care for the whole population of the mentally ill, was led by philanthropist and reformer Dorothea Dix (1971). The philosophy of care that drove and supported this reform effort was the "cult of curability," the view that mental illness was a response to toxic social conditions and could be cured by a therapeutic environment. This perspective was supported by the previous successes of the asylum. Under Dorothea Dix's leadership, asylums were established in twenty-eight of the existing thirty-three states.

Phase Two, 1840–1870: The Split Between Public and Private Psychiatry

Public sector involvement in psychiatric treatment began when the state provided the capital funds for the construction of the new hospitals, with local communities continuing to bear the responsibility for the cost of care of each patient admitted. The pattern for such state involvement was set in 1829 in Massachusetts when Horace Mann chaired a committee that recommended the development of the Worcester Lunatic Asylum, which was built in 1832. This step toward a publicly supported, as opposed to philanthropically supported, system represented the *first cost shift* in the institutional care of the mentally ill in the United States and was the step that ultimately separated the care of the well-off from the indigent and established the private and the public systems.

As the demand for institutional care continued to grow, the state-supported asylums began to be filled with increasingly chronic and impoverished patients (Deutsch, 1937). Patients from the more affluent families turned to private facilities for care, and increasingly, private resources were devoted to building facilities for paying patients. A two-class system was solidified, and from this point on, the public and private systems experienced relatively separate lines of development.

Phase Three, 1870–1940: The Mental Hygiene Movement and the Creation of the State Hospital

The separate development of public and private systems was largely reflected in the kinds of services each system provided.

Creation of State Mental Hospitals. The public asylums rapidly became filled beyond capacity, and beyond initial configurational expectations, with poor, lower-class patients. By the 1870s, the role of the state hospital in providing primarily custodial care and community protection was established, and treatment became of secondary importance. This very delimited view of the original functions of the psychiatric hospital (crisis control, acute treatment, rehabilitation, and custodial care) debilitated the role of the institution and led to increasingly widespread abuses. The quality of care deteriorated, access to facilities was severely limited due to overcrowding, and the costs of caring for the mentally ill in these facilities became unbearable for the local communities.

The identification and focus on these abuses in the U.S. system came both from groups such as those led by Dorothea Dix in the United States and from British psychiatrists, who attacked the support of this system by U.S. psychiatrists (Deutsch, 1944; Grob, 1983). The public outcry against the abuses led to an attempted resolution which entailed a shift in the social level of responsibility for running the asylums. The pattern was set by New York and Massachusetts (Grob, 1992) and was marked in 1890 by the New York State Care Act, which established the precedent for the state to assume full financial responsibility for the care and treatment of the mentally ill. This step represented the *second cost shift* in the care of the mentally ill, transferring the cost of care from local communities entirely to the state. As the control of the asylums shifted to the state, the designation of these institutions was changed from "asylum" to "state mental hospital."

It was thought that, by this cost shift, local communities' vested interests in not providing care, that is, in using prisons, or almshouses or various other institutions as alternatives to care, would be curtailed and the mentally ill poor could receive more appropriate and psychiatrically specific care. Further, with a less contentious, more stable single source of funding, it was felt that the conditions for care could be improved. What happened, however, was that the opportunity for cost shifting was exuberantly received by the local communities, and they rapidly took advantage of this windfall. Communities went beyond the intent of the law and passed along to the state, and to the asylum, care for a variety of individuals not originally conceived as falling under the act, such as the aged.

By 1910, under these changed conditions of funding, the number of psychiatric hospitals had grown from approximately 200 in 1875 to over 4,000 nationwide, and from 1903 to 1950, the number of patients in the state mental hospitals increased 240 percent, twice as much as the growth of the general population (Morrissey and Goldman, 1984). As might be expected given these conditions, problems of overcrowding occurred within the state-funded facilities. Cost containment led to low staffing and the general deterioration of the state hospitals into purely custodial institutions. In order to effect cost savings, the size of these institutions grew enormously, concomitantly worsening the problems of abuse. This ultimately led to the state of affairs known as "warehousing" of the mentally ill. Hence, although this cost shift relieved the community of the costs of the mentally ill, it did little to rectify the issues of quality or access, and in actuality, managed to shift the costs without reducing them.

The Mental Hygiene Movement and Psychopathic Hospitals. While this process was evolving on the public side, a different process was occurring on the private side, where the evolution of institutional care was heavily influenced by the initiation of a new movement in psychiatry by Clifford Beers. In 1908, Beers published the landmark book *A Mind That Found Itself* (Dain, 1980). The following year, Beers acquired the support of psychiatrist Adolf Meyer and psychologist and philosopher William James to help found the National Committee for Mental Hygiene. The mental hygiene movement arose as an antidote to the prevailing belief, developing because of the dominant picture of asylums and state hospitals as custodial care institutions, that mental illness was chronic and incurable. Beers's personal account of his own life was a dramatic statement to the contrary. His sentiment fit well with a new perspective in psychiatry embodied in the work of Adolf Meyer (1919), who laid the foundations for scientific psychiatry in the United States: "The psychiatrist may at last say that he has found himself. Instead of being singled out from the rest of physicians as what used to be called 'an asylum man,' pure and simple he has found his sphere in the special study of the *patient as a person*; the special study of the total activities and total behaviors, the kind of thing which cannot be singled out as merely the function of any one detachable organ, not even of the brain itself." This perspective firmly established the care of the mentally ill as a separate discipline and provided the necessary backdrop for research and knowledge to become the driving forces behind the changing nature of psychiatry.

The mental hygiene movement took concrete shape in various forms: one of the most relevant of these for institutional care was the concept of a "psychopathic hospital," that is, a hospital dedicated to acute treatment, rather than custodial care, and established in such a way that it was integrated with a university department of psychiatry. The goal of this concept was to implement a new scientific psychiatry and advance that field. Under this reform, various other alternative institutions supporting outpatient care, such as child guidance clinics and mental health agencies, were begun and new professions were developed. Thus, on the private side, the development of these new institutions, focused on acute care, led to the disaggregation of acute treatment from the custodial function, which was relegated largely to the state hospital.

Phase Four, 1940 to Present: Psychiatry as Science

The current period has been marked by the increasing disaggregation of the functions and locations of care. A growth in knowledge and technology in psychiatry was largely responsible for this process. As inpatient psychiatry found its niche, the function of the inpatient unit became increasingly restricted to crisis stabilization and acute treatment. Hence, the remaining functions of care, rehabilitation and custodial care, were either subsumed by other structures or neglected. On the private side, this disaggregation of the function and location of care was marked by the expansion of free-standing psychiatric hospitals, general hospital psychiatric units, and outpatient clinics. On the public side, it was marked by the advent of community mental health centers and the eventual development of community support programs.

Public System, 1940–1960: Community Mental Health Centers. The advent of World War II, the knowledge gained in psychiatric practice during that period, some key legislation immediately following the war, the increasing use of psychoanalysis, and the growth of general medical knowledge, greatly facilitated the development of more scientifically based psychiatry, and general hospital units, psychiatric outpatient clinics, and free-standing psychiatric hospitals grew substantially. Specific influences included the following:

During WWII, during which 12 of every 100 men examined were rejected for neuropsychiatric reasons and the number of medical officers assigned to psychiatry in the U.S. Army had to be increased from 25 to over 2,000, there was renewed interest in psychiatry and the treatment of mental illness (Szasz, 1970).

The Mental Health Services Act of 1946 greatly expanded the number of community-based psychiatrists, the number growing from about 3,500 in 1945 to about 25,000 in 1975 (Johnson, 1975).

Key legislation facilitated the construction of hospitals and units devoted to psychiatric care.

The growth of private insurance made funds available to support psychiatric care.

Additionally, the developing knowledge base lent credibility to treating mental illness in such settings. This knowledge included principles of care based on psychoanalysis; the emergence of psychopharmacology, which allowed rapid recuperation from illness and control of highly disturbed behavior; the introduction of the brief treatment techniques learned during World War II; and the expansion of the prevalence and technology of outpatient care.

As a result of these influences, a growth in alternative levels of care ensued. Before 1948, more than half of all states had no outpatient clinics. By 1949, all but five states had at least one. By 1955, there were over 1,200 outpatient psychiatric clinics, two-thirds of them supported or aided by states.

The explosion of knowledge and other concomitant factors resulted in an enormous growth in the psychiatric profession and a shift in treatment philosophy. Once again, the development of new knowledge and the shift in treatment philosophy coincided with growing concerns about cost and patient abuse, a concern that led to a radical shift in the structure of the mental health care delivery system. As we began to understand, again and anew, the "treatability" of mental illness and the value of alternative levels of care, the poor and often abusive conditions of the state facilities, the expenses of running these facilities, a concern about the institutionalization of the mentally ill (as a result of prolonged isolative and apathetic inpatient stays), and a greater emphasis on the rights of the mentally ill were all highlighted. Taken together, these factors argued against the psychiatric hospital as the ideal setting for effective treatment. The restructuring that followed was the process known as "deinstitutionalization."

Public System, 1960 to mid 1970s: Deinstitutionalization. Deinstitutionalization ultimately led to a major shift in the location of care. The explicit emphasis of deinstitutionalization and its concomitant support vehicle, the community mental health center (CMHC) movement, was to move the locus of care from a fixed institution into the community. This shift in the location of treatment, deriving from the factors noted earlier, was supported by a growing knowledge base of "social psychiatry." The development of empirical information regarding the influence of a broad range of social variables on mental health and mental illness lent force to a strong momentum for movement of patients from inpatient care facilities to a setting of stimulation, rehabilitation, enfranchisement, and reengagement in the mainstream of life. This process was supported by several major political actions.

Once again, New York State played a leading role, enacting, in 1954, the Community Mental Health Services Act, which provided for expansion of outpatient treatment. California, shortly thereafter, passed the Short-Doyle Act, a similar measure that increased state-funding for outpatient clinics. These actions were supported by the National Institute of Mental Health (NIMH) at a federal level. The deinstitutionalization process was further supported at a federal level by the 1955 final report to the Joint Commission on Mental Illness and Health, *Action for Mental Health*, and the subsequent passage of the Community Mental Health Services Act of 1961. Concomitantly, the passage of Medicaid and Medicare legislation in 1963 enabled the movement of aged people from state hospitals into nursing homes (Morrissey and Goldman, 1984).

All of these forces permitted a major shift in location of care. However, this process also engendered the *third cost shift*, this one from the states to the federal government. Strong support could be found at the state legislative level for deinstitutionalization because of the availability of new federal funding. Following the federal legislation, there was a massive nationwide facilitation of the deinstitutionalization process. In 1955, there were 559,000 resident patients in state mental hospitals. By 1977, this number had fallen to 160,000 (Docherty, 1984). What is reflected in these numbers is that the type of care rendered by the state hospitals also shifted from custodial care to become more concordant with the focus of treatment at the private hospitals, that is, crisis stabilization and acute treatment. For example, the total number of episodes of care in 1955 and 1968 were very close. In 1955, 818,832 episodes of care occurred in state hospitals; in 1968, 791,819 (Grob, 1992). However, the nature of care differed dramatically, resulting in a much lower daily resident census in later years. For example, the average mid 1950s length of stay of six months, had fallen to three weeks by the mid 1970s. In this process, we developed a de facto system in which acute care was provided both at the local level and at the state hospital level.

Unfortunately, although the goal of the deinstitutionalization movement was to provide necessary care for the mentally ill through a community-based system, to a large extent this was not the role adopted by the CMHCs. The CMHCs were unprepared for the massive influx of severely disturbed patients, with a wide diversity of needs, released from the state hospitals; additionally, despite having to serve a larger proportion of the mentally ill, the CMHCs received insufficient funding; and finally, the focus of these centers was largely on the prevention of chronicity and the application of brief treatments for the acutely ill, which led to a large population of chronically mentally ill "failures" from the previous system remaining untreated. Hence, although the functions of crisis care, acute treatment, and to some extent rehabilitation were provided for, lacking in this scenario were clear and careful planning for custodial care and acceptable accommodations for individuals requiring a long-term protective environment.

Public System, 1975 to Present: Community Support Programs. In response to the lack of a system to adequately care for the chronically mentally ill, the National Institute of Mental Health launched the Community Support Program, which was designed to provide services uniquely suited for this population. This program, solidified by the *National Plan for the Chronically Mentally Ill* (1980) and the Mental Health Systems Act of 1980, was intended to support systems that ensured direct care and rehabilitation of the chronically mentally ill. Specific services that were funded included crisis care services, psychosocial rehabilitation services, supportive living and working arrangements, and case management services (Tessler and Goldman, 1982).

The Community Support Program was unique in two respects. First, it represented the first effort to reenfranchise the chronically mentally ill whose needs had largely been neglected by other reform efforts. This was important for a number of reasons. Prior to this time, the chronically mentally ill were regarded by some ideologues as patients who simply did not exist in large numbers and by cynics as patients who did not need and would not benefit from treatment. Neither of these views was a viable construct of the reality of mental illness, and neither allowed for an appropriate and humane response to this population's needs. Chronic mental illness is not rare, it is treatable, and there is hope for significant functional and symptomatological improvement in this population. In fact, society pays far more, socially and fiscally, for not appropriately treating this population than it does to develop and provide services and systems to meet this population's needs.

Fiscally, the National Advisory Mental Health Council has estimated the direct costs of treating chronic mental illness at approximately $20 billion per year. Indirect costs due to lost productivity, social welfare payments, criminal justice expenses, and so forth, however, amount to at least $48 billion per year. Additionally, it is estimated that a 10 percent increase in funds available for direct treatment would result in a 10 percent decrease in indirect costs—translating into an annual savings of $2.2 billion. Clearly, it is financially advisable to treat this population (National Advisory Mental Health Council, 1993).

Socially, a failure to adequately serve the chronically mentally ill perpetuates the stigma of mental illness and creates a second class of citizens who are denied necessary and beneficial services because of the nature of their illness.

The second unique aspect of the Community Support Program was that it focused not on the development of new locations of care, or new services, per se, but on a *system to coordinate* these services in a manner that would allow a less fragmented, more comprehensive, and continuous treatment process. Unfortunately, economic concerns once again interfered with the success of the reform efforts, and to date, the chronically mentally ill remain neglected and inadequately cared for.

Private System, 1960 to Present. The substantial reduction in state-run hospitals resulted in an increased demand for alternative accommodations for previously institutionalized patients for whom the CMHCs were not able to provide an adequate level of services. Additionally, the willingness of Medicaid, Medicare, and private insurers to reimburse for services provided at private institutions increased the profitability of these facilities. In fact, while the use of medical/surgical care became increasingly restricted by the amounts of prospective reimbursement and by diagnosis-related groups (DRGs), mental health care was characterized by continued charge- or cost-based reimbursement. Also, a 300 percent increase in the number of mental health professionals between 1955 and 1983, coupled with the elimination of state-level certificate-of-need programs, made the acquisition of the necessary resources to build and operate a psychiatric facility a relatively simple process (Duhl and Cummings, 1987). The interaction of the increased demand, increased supply, and increased profitability inevitably resulted in a massive expansion in the privatization of mental health care. From 1984 to 1988, the number of private psychiatric hospitals nearly doubled, to 381, and continued to grow. Additionally, the number of private psychiatric beds went from accounting for only 7 percent of total beds in 1970 to 35 percent in 1986 (Herrington, 1989).

The rapid growth of this intensive and expensive treatment alternative is very likely one of the primary reasons behind the percentage increase of mental health treatment costs, which have risen 2.5 times general medical inflation (Herrington, 1989). Indeed, mental health care has become unsustainably expensive. In 1990, the direct costs of treating mental illness were estimated at $67 billion, and the total costs of mental illness $148 billion. Costs for inpatient psychiatric care accounted for more than 60 percent of the direct treatment costs (National Advisory Mental Health Council, 1993).

The chronically mentally ill were often excluded from private facilities due to lack of available funds. Hence, their needs continued to be unmet. The private side, in effect, further shifted the cost and the responsibility for the chronically mentally ill into the public sector. The chronically mentally ill, simply by reason of insurance benefit design, became insurance indigents and thereby were converted to public sector patients, reinforcing the introduction of the second-class citizen view of the mentally ill and deepening the stigma surrounding their illnesses.

Furthermore, although the private sector has until recently enjoyed a relatively smooth period of expansion and growth, for the first time it has experienced a major scandal, mirroring the process of cost-abuse-scandal-reform on the public side and ultimately leading to a massive drive for reform. This scandal centered on allegations made against a major for-profit publicly held hospital chain. A full-scale government investigation probed allegations of false medical claims, conspiracy, kickbacks, and fraud against Medicare, Medicaid, and the Pentagon's insurance plan. Additionally, a consortium of thirteen insurance carriers brought a suit against the company for alleged billing fraud. The insurers alleged that the psychiatric hospitals were milking psychiatric patients' insurance coverage for profit by misrepresenting symptoms, billing for services not rendered, and other methods. These events led to reform not only within this specific corporation, but within the private inpatient psychiatric industry as a whole (Associated Press, 1993).

Although the reform efforts have been partially regulatory, they have largely taken the form of massive cost controls. These cost controls came largely in the form of reduced coverage for care and increasingly restrictive admission and utilization criteria. Specific attention has been placed on reducing the utilization of inpatient care, as this sector experienced the largest cost inflations. The most visible of these efforts was the introduction of managed care.

As a result of these cost and utilization controls, we have recently witnessed the disaggregation of the final functions of inpatient care—the separation of acute treatment from crisis intervention. The current era is thus marked by the provision of the four functions of care in several separate locations, with only crisis intervention remaining at the heart of the psychiatric hospital. Thus, inpatient psychiatrists must learn new, specific skills related to rapid symptom stabilization and treatment planning. Such skills were unnecessary in an era when the crisis could "take care of itself" because the focus was on acute treatment and time was available to complete the tasks of that treatment. Indeed, when the focus is on acute treatment and the time is present to permit such treatment, a crisis by and large does take care of itself. However, the costs and other pressures in contemporary psychiatry noted above have now moved us to a specific focus on crisis intervention as an essential area of clinical expertise and focus.

Phase Five: Where Will We Go from Here?

From a historical perspective, the trajectory of inpatient psychiatry as a whole is clear. As a consequence, we might expect that the next phase will push us toward moving crisis intervention out of the institutional setting. Indeed, there are many programs in this country already in place which carry out the crisis intervention function in the patient's home through the use of emergency intervention teams. If such a process should prove feasible, then the last vestige of the key functions of care will be removed from the institutional setting. If this is the case, we must ask: What will become of inpatient psychiatry? and, What is the appropriate reform effort that will end this cycle of knowledge growth, cost-shifting, abuse, and expose of abuses, that has, as of yet, failed to develop a system able to adequately care for the mentally ill?

Unfortunately, to date, despite the myriad changes and improvements in both the private and community systems, the needs of the mentally ill continue to be largely unmet or ignored. As has been the case historically, the uncoordinated growth of the current public and private psychiatric systems has resulted in continuing problems of cost, access, and quality. There has been an inevitable increase in mental health costs due to large systemic inefficiencies, large populations of mentally ill still not receiving appropriate treatment, and a cottage industry structure of care that isolates each clinician's resources, skills, and knowledge, thus making it difficult for any one patient to receive a full range of appropriate treatments.

These events have inevitably led to a mandate for reform. However, we are at a uniquely opportune point in history, as both the private and public sectors of mental health care struggle once again to reform the overall system. We therefore have the unique opportunity to rectify the situation we created 200 years ago, by rejoining the private and public sectors to form a unified, coordinated, and comprehensive system of care designed to meet the needs of all of the mentally ill.

Redefining the Psychiatric Health Care System

At its inception, the asylum fulfilled three main needs: the provision of services, a place for these services, and the coordination of these services. Despite the problems of these early asylums, they had one major advantage, namely, the provision of the full range of services in a single location. The major impact of the evolution in mental health care on the use of inpatient psychiatry in the United States has been, as described earlier, to disaggregate the complex set of functions (crisis intervention, treatment of the acute episode of illness, rehabilitation from that acute episode, and if necessary, custodial care) that were originally assigned to institutionally based psychiatric care and to distribute these functions to separate locations for care. This process of separation has been gradual and progressive. Initially, there was a separation of the custodial function from the three treatment functions. Then, with the growth of outpatient care, various rehabilitative functions were separated. Finally, with the growth of managed care and other regulatory agencies, the separation of acute treatment and crisis intervention occurred.

As we have disaggregated the functions of care and their locations, we have expanded the mental health care system while simultaneously losing a great deal that the original psychiatric inpatient setting provided on its own. We have dissected the whole without proper regard for the preservation of its integrity. Therefore, perhaps it is not so odd that the key to a successful reform, one that provides high quality, affordable, and accessible care, may be to ensure that each of the primary tasks of the early asylum is carried out.

By disaggregating the functions of care and abandoning the psychiatric hospital as the primary location for the provision of all of these functions, we have created environments that have become progressively dependent on communication systems, organizational structures, and coordinating entities that simply do not exist. Our primary challenge today is to finally develop a mental health care *system* that truly controls costs, ensures access, and provides quality care.

The general shape that a reformed system of mental health care should take is reasonably clear. The first and most essential element of such a reform is that we should have a one-class system. That is, health care reform should provide a sufficient benefit structure for public sector care. This would be beneficial in the following ways: it would reduce the stigma of chronic mental illness that is associated with simply being a public sector patient; it would serve to broaden societal concern with the provision of care made available to the chronically mentally ill, by yoking all members of society to a similar benefit structure; and it would diminish the erroneous and maladaptive belief that has characterized our mental health care system for almost 200 years, that the chronically mentally ill could be taken care of somewhere else and paid for by someone else.

The second major element of a reformed mental health care system is a new conceptualization of our mental health care system. The system that has characterized mental health care was conceived in terms of a "continuum of care." This continuum was defined by a number of treatment programs, which varied in their ability to provide effective interventions for increasingly severely disturbed psychiatric patients. Generally, the continuum included outpatient, partial hospital, residential, and inpatient care. Over the years, a number of additional treatment services have been added, but all of them are conceived as points along a unidimensional continuum of care.

However, as the history of change in institutional psychiatric care has revealed, patient care services are not intrinsically linked to the location of care. Once we separate service and location, it becomes clear that, in fact, there is not a single continuum of care in which treatment location and clinical services covary, but rather two continua: a continuum of locations and a continuum of clinical services. These continua constitute a matrix of care.

In our current system, intensity of setting and intensity of clinical services are linked and covary. In other words, individuals who need a lot of clinical services routinely receive them in the most restrictive environment. Hence, the acutely psychotic patient is relegated to the inpatient setting.

But the matrix formed by the two continua demonstrates that there are a number of potential combinations of settings and clinical services that our current system cannot offer. There are patients who require intensive clinical services but only minimal environmental support, such as victims of acute trauma who may require family, group, and individual therapy. There are also patients, such as chronic schizophrenic patients, maintained in a community program who suffer relapse to an acute psychotic decompensation and who require an intense treatment setting yet only infrequent, limited clinical services. If these options are not provided, patients are forced either to pay for unnecessary services or to receive an inadequate level of care.

There are at least two advantages to the matrix conceptualization. First, it allows independent variation of the intensity of treatment setting and of clinical services to meet the needs of an individual patient; in other words, it allows us to mix and match treatment settings and clinical services to achieve the most efficient combination. Second, it allows much greater latitude in developing and designing innovative, cost-effective treatment "products" geared to the special needs of each individual.

Developing such a matrix of care does not involve the creation of several new treatments, or facilities for those treatments, but rather calls for the effective organization and systematization of the locations and services currently available. Such a system would dissolve the historical separation of the public and private sectors and would strategically develop a matrix of care for each community, one that involved the services and locations traditionally provided by each sector.

A prerequisite to the effective implementation of a matrix of care is the effective coordination of the range of services and settings. It is with regard to the coordination of service that the inpatient psychiatric setting may still have its most influential and important role to play in the future of mental health care. In addition to a restricted range of services, the role of a coordinating center for the matrix of care might well fall to inpatient psychiatric programs. In any case, at this point in our history, the role of inpatient psychiatry has changed and is changing radically. Below, I discuss the current and past issues that I feel an inpatient psychiatric setting must address in order to successfully adapt to the present and future.

Redefining the Role of the Inpatient Facility

Three issues have remained constant as our society's goals for an adequate and acceptable health care system: reasonable cost, high quality, and broad access to care. These three issues have been greatly highlighted and invigorated by the contemporary focus on health care reform. The beauty of this is that these same issues lend measurable goals to today's health care reform efforts, that is, reduced cost, improved quality, and increased access.

None of the reform efforts enacted to date have truly resolved the issues of cost, quality, and access that have plagued the U.S. health care system. As noted earlier, the introduction of a matrix conceptualization and the dissolution of the traditional public/private boundaries will do much to rectify some of these issues. However, a historical review further reveals that this failure to resolve these issues may depend on the extent to which each reform effort has not appropriately focused on the systemic issues that affect cost, quality, and access. Specifically, none of the historical reform efforts has adequately focused on the transfer of knowledge from research into practice to ensure state-of-the-art, high-quality care; on the generation of practical research to guide clinical and policy decisions regarding the effectiveness and efficiency of specific services and delivery systems; and on the destigmatization of mental illness, to ensure that the full range of the mentally ill, especially the chronically mentally ill, are provided with appropriate care in appropriate locations, that is, not in almshouses, jails, or nursing homes.

The challenge to the mental health care system is to enact a reform that will ensure the mentally ill receive high-quality, affordable, and accessible care. This goal can be realized if we ensure the availability of appropriate treatment services and settings for the functions of crisis intervention, treatment, rehabilitation, and asylum; support the development of a system for the coordination of this care; and address the three systemic issues discussed here, in order to ensure that the reform is conducted in an empirically sound and informed manner.

The inpatient psychiatric center can play an influential and important role in this new system. Today, inpatient psychiatry is only responsible for providing *some* psychiatric services and *some* of the necessary locations of care. Its role in the actual provision of services has been diminished, rightfully so, as we have come to recognize that treatment can be provided in many places and that the selection of place can be used as a therapeutic instrument in order to enhance the well-being of the patient and reduce costs to the system. However, the need for inpatient psychiatry once again to assume responsibility for the coordination of care, as it implicitly did in the early days of the asylum, has never been greater. Fortunately, the psychiatric hospital remains uniquely suited to fulfill this task.

Assuming the New Role

There are two major functions that inpatient psychiatry will serve in the future: a clinical service function and a coordination-of-care function. The latter function, as I have mentioned, represents a relatively new role for the inpatient setting and has been developing in a somewhat haphazard fashion—some institutions are much further advanced than others in supporting the development of this function. I will discuss each of these functions in turn.

Clinical Function. Direct clinical services at the inpatient setting in the foreseeable future will be diminished relative to the last ten years. However, a variety of practical issues make it likely that for the next ten years, the following clinical functions will characterize inpatient psychiatric care:

Crisis intervention. The principle clinical function of inpatient psychiatry will be to provide protection, risk reduction, and symptom stabilization over very short periods of time to patients who are experiencing an acute crisis. This will be an active area of education and clinical development. New programs, methodologies, and technologies will be developed to improve and refine the skillful application of this crisis intervention function.

Complex diagnostic assessment. There will be some patients who will continue to present a complicated diagnostic problem, such as the patient whose symptoms may be of a complicated medical or neurological origin or of an unusual symptomatic distribution. The necessity for multiple diagnostic tests and the coordination of the resulting information may simply make this process more efficient if it is carried out as part of an organized, institutionally based diagnostic program.

Specialized treatment. There are two categories of patients who will still differentially benefit from inpatient treatment. These are, first, patients with relatively standard diagnoses who have not responded to standard treatment and are reflecting a deteriorating course of illness. The twenty-four-hour observation afforded by the inpatient setting, with its ability to reveal symptoms or other clues that may not have been accessible in outpatient settings and to ensure the delivery of treatment, make the inpatient setting useful for serving this type of patient. Second, patients with specific complicated problems such as comorbid substance abuse disorder or dissociative disorder in the context of a destructive living situation, and those who require multiple treatments simultaneously delivered in a coordinated fashion or whose treatment courses may be expected to present episodes of risk or require a specialized therapeutic environment for the delivery of the treatment, such as high-risk medication protocols, will also require the presence of highly specialized treatment programs in inpatient settings.

These relatively high-tech functions of the inpatient unit, however, will represent only a small part of clinical activity and, if reform proceeds properly, a much smaller part of the mental health care dollar. The major function of inpatient units of today will likely switch to the second function, the coordination of care.

Coordination of Care. The inpatient psychiatric facility is one of the few entities in the current mental health system which, by and large, continues to hold the critical mass of resources (personnel, space, equipment) necessary to carry out the task of coordination. This coordination will have two aspects. The first is to effectively accomplish the coordination of setting and service to provide for crisis intervention, treatment, rehabilitation, and asylum, a task that previously was not accomplished. The second is to address the three specific tasks necessary for an adequate system of care, which I mentioned earlier, namely, knowledge transfer, the generation of new practical knowledge, and the reversal of stigma.

Coordination of Treatment Services. We have historically failed to recognize the essential need for a coordinating entity in psychiatry. In its initial form, the asylum was well suited to this task and assumed it perhaps without even realizing its importance. However, as location and function become separated from a central entity, the task of coordination becomes both more difficult and more necessary. By historically failing to address the chronic and recurring nature of mental illness, we have left the majority of seriously ill patients without adequate care. Our emphasis has, during this last epoch, been on acute treatment, and we have behaved as though, if we could only find the silver bullet, our problems would be solved. In essence, we deluded ourselves into believing that mental illness could be cured if only we could find the right treatment. The fact is, however, that the provision of a discrete psychiatric service, with no coordinated services before or after a specific intervention, regardless of its excellence, does not effectively address the needs of the mentally ill. Today, with the shift of direct clinical activity in the inpatient setting from treatment to crisis intervention, this issue assumes an intense urgency. The psychiatric hospital must shift its emphasis from provider of care to coordinator of care.

Coordination of Knowledge Generation, Transfer, and Dissemination. There is a problem of ignorance, also called the knowledge gap problem, that has troubled mental health care for an extended period. On the nonprofessional side, it appears in the misassumptions and prejudices that the general public holds about mental illness. On the professional side, it appears in the overly long lag time between the development of new knowledge and the transformation and introduction of this new knowledge into practice.

Dissemination of new knowledge into practice. There is currently no effective process of knowledge transfer. The NIMH has repeatedly noted that it takes approximately ten to fifteen years for new knowledge to become fully integrated into practice. This time delay is unacceptable in an era in which new effective treatments are available and are desperately needed by our patients. The flaws in the organization of the mental health system have directly contributed to this delay. At one end, we have the academic system, which is primarily concerned with basic knowledge and research; at the other end, we have a private practice system structured as a cottage-industry and concerned almost entirely with delimited ranges of direct patient care. No institution has stood in the middle to rapidly teach and utilize the advances in knowledge that occur. The psychiatric hospital has the potential to become the missing intermediary institution required to alleviate this problem.

Generation of practical knowledge. New scientific knowledge in mental health care has been generated, for the most part, in university settings. The prestige structure of universities has tended to direct most of this knowledge generation activity into basic science studies. This has left us with a progressively untenable state of affairs. For example, for twenty years there were two antidepressants used to treat most depressed patients: amitriptyline and imipramine. Yet we had no knowledge regarding which patients would differentially respond to one or the other, if there was such differential response, and what was the likely course if there was no response to the one being used first. Such a study can only feasibly be done with very large numbers of patients. The implication is that clinical settings would be needed to carry out such studies. Yet our clinical settings have not been organized to do such work. Psychiatric inpatient settings are uniquely suited to become the coordinating centers to conduct such practical research to answer many important clinical and operational questions.

In addition to addressing the efficacy of specific treatments, the incidence and likelihood of acquiring low-frequency side effects, and so forth, the opportunity exists for research to address less traditional but critically important questions for health care systems management. Specifically, the development of the pragmatic research function within clinical settings can greatly expand the efficiency and effectiveness of care. It will allow us to measure the effectiveness of different health care structures, different clinical management systems, and administrative policies and procedures on treatment outcome. Additionally, the effect of provider type, staffing models, and different administrative, financial, or educational incentives can be examined objectively. This information is essential to rational health services planning. The successful inpatient settings of the future will include the capacity to facilitate such work.

Dissemination of new knowledge to the community and the reversal of stigma. Based in ignorance, a type of prejudice, worse than the type previously associated with such medical illnesses as cancer, continues to further burden and increase the suffering of the mentally ill. Most regrettably, it keeps many people who could be effectively helped by today's treatments from receiving that help. The U.S. public continues to hold erroneous and maladaptive beliefs about the mentally ill. According to a survey conducted by the Robert Wood Johnson Program on Chronic Mental Illness, only one in four Americans is very well informed about mental illness, 61 percent feel mental illness could be caused by a lack of discipline, one in four believes the chronically mentally ill are more dangerous than the general population, and 26 percent believe that mental illness can never really be cured (Borinstein, 1992).

Such beliefs are born in ignorance and bred by fear. A constant active program of effective community education, involving substantial personal contact both with spokespersons for the mentally ill and professionals skilled in working with the mentally ill in alleviating psychological distress, is needed to change this now archaic and destructive state of ignorance and system of beliefs. Once again, the inpatient psychiatry facility has the resources available to engage in and conduct such activity. Short-sighted concerns regarding the cost of such work serve to undermine the viability of that institution in its own local setting and the likelihood that, nationwide, the mentally ill will receive appropriate care. A key task of inpatient psychiatric units in their role as coordinators of care is to conduct active, ongoing, and continuous programs of community education.

Conclusion

Viewed in its most positive light, the current state of affairs in inpatient psychiatry represents an opportunity of enormous historical magnitude. This is the opportunity to bring to fruition a process which has been unfolding over the last two centuries. This process has been to disaggregate, define, and refine the core services that need to be provided to ensure a comprehensive system of care for the mentally ill and to elaborate a variety of settings in which this care can be administered most effectively and most efficiently. The growth in scientific knowledge regarding treatment and the enormous growth in the capacity to provide organized systems of communication and information processing now make it possible to provide a truly comprehensive matrix of care for the mentally ill that is empirically grounded and informed by the latest knowledge.

Another major aspect of the historical unfolding over the last two centuries is the gradual spreading of the costs of caring for the mentally ill through the entirety of our society—from the local communities to states to the federal government on the public side, and from private individuals to private employers and employees on the private side. We now have the opportunity to bring that process, also, to full fruition in the development of a truly adequate, compulsory benefit package as part of health care reform. The availability, for the first time, of such a source of adequate and appropriate funding has the potential to usher in an era unprecedented in our history.

This is the context in which inpatient psychiatry is practiced today. I have discussed this context because it is important in framing and understanding the place and utility of the specific functions which now characterize, and very likely will continue to characterize, the clinical activity of the psychiatric inpatient program. It is to these clinical activities that the remainder of this volume is dedicated. Additionally, it is hoped that the remaining chapters will help those responsible for the development and management of inpatient programs to plan effectively for the future.

References

Associated Press. "NME to Pay Insurers $89 Million to Settle Fraud Suit." *Dallas Morning News,* Dec. 14, 1993.

Borinstein, A. M. "Public Attitudes Toward Persons with Mental Illness." *Health Affairs,* 1992, *11,* 186–196.

Dain, N. *Clifford W. Beers: Advocate for the Insane.* Pittsburgh, Penn.: University of Pittsburgh Press, 1980.

Deutsch, A. *The Mentally Ill in America: A History of Their Care and Treatment from Colonial Times.* New York: Columbia University Press, 1937.

Deutsch, A. "The History of Mental Hygiene." In J. K. Hall, G. Zilboorg, and H. A. Bunker (eds.), *One Hundred Years of American Psychiatry.* New York: Columbia University Press, 1944.

Dix, D. *On Behalf of the Insane Poor: Selected Reports* (reprint). New York: Arno Press, 1971.

Docherty, J. P. "We Turned the Mentally Ill into the Streets." *Newsday,* Dec. 2, 1984, pp. 9–10.

Duhl, L. J., and Cummings, N. A. *The Future of Mental Health Services.* New York: Springer, 1987.

Grob, G. N. *Mental Illness and American Society, 1875–1940.* Princeton, N.J.: Princeton University Press, 1983.

Grob, G. N. "Mental Health Policy in America: Myths and Realities." *Health Affairs,* Fall 1992, pp. 7–22.

Herrington, B. S. "Outpatient Managed Care Inevitable." *Psychiatric News,* Nov. 3, 1989, pp. 16–22.

Johnson, J. C. "The Future of Psychiatry in General Hospitals." *Psychiatric Annals,* 1975, *5,* 37–55.

Meyer, A. *Adolf Meyer Papers.* Baltimore, Md.: Chesney Medical Archives, Johns Hopkins Medical Institutions, 1919.

Morrissey, J. P., and Goldman, H. H. "Cycles of Reform in the Care of the Chronically Mentally Ill." *Hospital and Community Psychiatry,* 1984, *35,* 785–793.

National Advisory Mental Health Council. "Health Care Reform for Americans with Severe Mental Illness." *American Journal of Psychiatry,* 1993, *150* (10), 1447–1465.

National Plan for the Chronically Mentally Ill: Final Draft Report to the Secretary of Health and Human Services. Washington, D.C.: Department of Health and Human Services, 1980.

Szasz, T. S. *The Manufacture of Madness.* New York: HarperCollins, 1970.

Tessler, R. C., and Goldman, H. H. *The Chronically Mentally Ill: Assessing the Community Support Programs.* Cambridge, Mass.: Ballinger, 1982.

JOHN P. DOCHERTY, M.D., is professor of clinical psychiatry and medical director of the Mental Health Group at the University of California, Los Angeles.

An examination of the impact of managed behavioral care programs on psychiatry emphasizes efforts to manage variability in treatment approach and describes three distinct generations of programs.

The Emergence of Managed Care and Its Impact on Psychiatry

John Bartlett

The challenges of working within a managed care environment have become a daily reality for virtually every psychiatrist and psychiatric hospital throughout the country. Few and far between are those markets where there is no managed care presence; in fact, the opposite is much more likely to be the case, with multiple managed care vendors operating in any given location. It is becoming increasingly clear that delivery of mental health and substance abuse care has entered what some are calling the era of managed care.

The available data on managed care's growth and its impact on the delivery of psychiatric and substance abuse care in this country support this impression. The Foster Higgins health care benefits survey of employers for 1992 revealed that, of the 1,700 firms responding, 83 percent had a requirement for precertification of inpatient care, 66 percent required ongoing review of inpatient care, and 69 percent provided for case management of catastrophic cases. In addition, almost one in four employers in 1992 was using a specialty behavioral care vendor to provide this oversight, an increase of 40 percent over the reported use of such vendors the previous year (J. Foster Higgins, 1992). From the providers' point of view, the 1993 survey on psychiatric utilization conducted by the National Association of Psychiatric Health Systems through its member organizations revealed a continued increase in the prevalence and impact of managed mental health care on providers' operations. The association's members reported, for example, that, in 1992, 64 percent of all patient admissions required prior outside review, and 70 percent of these patients required outside review to extend their stays. Overall, 94 percent of the survey respondents reported that the impact of outside utilization management activities on their operations had increased over the prior twelve months (National Association of Psychiatric Health Systems, 1993).

This chapter will examine the forces that have led to this growth in managed behavioral care programs, the impact these programs have had on inpatient psychiatry, and the developmental course of these programs.

The Case for Managed Care

In the face of such growing influence, it would seem wise to ask, What has ushered in this era of managed care? What forces led to its creation, contributed to its rapid growth, and shaped its development? It is my belief, both from my clinical experience as a psychiatrist and my ten-year career within managed care, that the growth and current influence of managed care are the direct result of the failures of the previous unmanaged fee-for-service system (or rather, nonsystem) to address adequately the concerns of a variety of legitimate stockholders. These concerns include, among others, the needs of patients, the perceptions of payers, and the tools and techniques of providers. Let us examine each of these areas briefly.

In the first area, that of patients' needs, there is irrefutable evidence for the existence of significant demand for mental health and substance abuse services. The Epidemiological Catchment Area Survey of the National Institute of Mental Health explored the prevalence of serious mental illness and substance abuse throughout the United States. Using sound survey techniques, Myers and his coinvestigators (1984) were able to demonstrate a six-month prevalence rate for major psychiatric disorders of 15 percent and a lifetime prevalence rate for these same conditions of over 25 percent. In addition to this identified need, there is compelling evidence that there exists in the primary care setting a large, often unrecognized, and usually inappropriately treated group of mental health and substance abuse patients (Eisenberg, 1992). And finally, from a less scientific but no less convincing point of view, there is the daily litany of concerns that confront all of us about the homeless, drugs, and the problems of adolescents, including suicide and violence. Repeatedly, through the media as well as through our own experiences, these problems make their presence known.

Yet demand alone does not adequately, or even appropriately, define the full range of the needs and expectations of our patients. There exist other criteria by which both potential and actual consumers of mental health and substance abuse services value our services, and in these other areas, we are often poorly informed and even inattentive. For example, patients with resources (that is, either insurance or disposable income) find themselves confronted with an oftentimes bewildering array of treatment resources and approaches. Moreover, in the face of this wide variability and set of choices, they often receive little to no assistance in making informed choices as to the "best" treatment. At worst, patients are confronted with what sometimes has seemed like a concerted effort to promote what one author has called the "equivalency of therapies" myth (Giles, 1991).

Even individuals whose mental status in no way precludes them from making informed choices in other areas of their lives are most often not interacted with as equals or partners in the treatment process but rather as recipients of dictates from on high about both what ails them and what to do about it. This hierarchical, illness-oriented approach to many problems has frequently led our customers to the conclusion that the system and the providers in it are unresponsive to their needs and concerns. In fact, there is extensive research that demonstrates the often wide discrepancies between patient and therapist expectations of the treatment process (Garfield, 1986). Even more disturbing is the fact that patients without resources have often found themselves without access to needed care and qualified providers, especially psychiatrists.

The unmanaged fee-for-service system also failed to adequately address the concerns of payers. In the face of a perception of rapidly escalating costs for mental health and chemical dependency care, payers became increasingly troubled by the wide variability in treatment approaches and the expense they experienced in the marketplace. They also became concerned over time with the lack of accountability they saw on the part of many providers. This lack of accountability took many forms, but a particularly troubling one was what I call treatment planning by benefit design, in which providers would seem to develop their specific approaches to any given patient according to the number of inpatient days or outpatient visits that individual had in his or her benefit package. Under this approach, when the benefits were exhausted, the need for treatment would disappear, only to resurface later when the patient's benefits were reactivated, or in the case of patients who had reached their lifetime limits of coverage, further treatment would be provided in a public facility. This perception on the part of many private payers of providers' treatment planning by benefit design, coupled with the perception of escalating costs, led many payers to adopt benefit restriction as a legitimate risk management strategy. Such benefit restriction can take many forms, such as lower coinsurance rates for mental health and chemical dependency treatment, higher deductibles, exclusion from catastrophic coverage, and separate and lower lifetime maximums. In all of these, the intent is to limit the financial exposure of the payer and therefore to limit the payer's risk.

As clinicians, however, we recognize that such an approach, although financially sound, quickly becomes clinically bankrupt by creating benefit designs that are severely limited or that do not cover all appropriate levels of care. The old, unmanaged fee-for-service system, then, failed providers as well by driving their treatment options in directions or to degrees that were clinically inappropriate. In its most flagrant form, this failure has taken the form of frank discrimination against mental health and chemical dependency treatments and on occasion has even led to open discussion of complete elimination of benefits in these areas.

Because of these very real failures of an unmanaged, fee-for-service approach, it is a fallacy to see the growth and influence of managed behavioral care as being primarily cost driven. While concerns about cost certainly have played and continue to play a role, they do so in the context of a search for value on the part of most organizations that have adopted a managed behavioral care program. These organizations uniformly, in my experience, recognize the importance of providing for an appropriate level of mental health and chemical dependency benefits in their health benefits programs. However, as prudent purchasers of a variety of goods and services, they also want to better understand the interplay between the costs they are bearing and the quality of what they are paying for, with particular attention to the results of the treatments and services provided.

In short, managed behavioral care has risen to the position of prominence it occupies in today's health care marketplace because the perceived value of the care being purchased under the old system was no longer clearly worth the cost to those paying the bills. In the context of this failure, managed care (or perhaps more accurately, the management of care at the level of the delivery system) has represented the best vehicle for addressing the variety of failures outlined here, providing the opportunity for reasonable and effective care at a sustainable cost. In fact, it may well represent the last and best alternative to the approach of benefit restriction or elimination, which is only concerned with cost.

Theoretical Foundations

How does managed care address the failures of the unmanaged fee-for-service program? It does so by administering mental health and chemical dependency benefits through the determination of the medical appropriateness of individual treatment plans. Rather than relying on benefit design alone to determine what is covered in any given situation, it relies on judgments of the adequacy, relevance, and effectiveness of proposed treatment approaches. If one thinks of a typology that dichotomizes change into revolutionary (radical, turbulent, discontinuous) and evolutionary (gradual, incremental) categories, it becomes clear that there is nothing revolutionary about this approach (Bartlett, 1993). It merely represents an extension of the medical-surgical reimbursement system that applies both benefit design (what is covered) and determinations of clinical appropriateness (when it is covered) in making determinations of financial responsibility under group benefit plans. For example, most if not all such plans provide coverage for surgical treatment of diseases of the gall bladder and common bile duct; yet none provide for payment for such surgery in the absence of appropriate clinical indications, such as right upper quadrant pain, nausea, and vomiting, among others. In a similar fashion, under a managed care approach, the benefit design certainly allows for inpatient hospitalization, often at more generous levels or with less financial impact on the covered individual than traditional indemnity plans. However, these benefits are only covered in the presence of appropriate clinical indications and for only so long as these indications continue to exist.

What is revolutionary, and therefore the cause of much discussion, disagreement, and even turbulence, is that managed behavioral care limits the scope of these clinical indications and therefore what is defined as medically appropriate. This limitation of scope is a significant and discontinuous change from what was allowed under the old, unmanaged fee-for-service system and flies squarely in the face of the "equivalency of therapies" myth discussed earlier, where wide variations in treatment approach and indications were tolerated. In a strategic sense, then, managed behavioral care is an attempt to reduce variability in the treatment of mental health and substance abuse conditions.

Moreover, in seeking such reductions in the breadth and scope of appropriate care, managed behavioral care has been guided by a clear and explicit set of principles. These include considerations of effectiveness, or the ability to produce the desired result; efficiency, or the production of that result with minimal waste; and empirical support for statements of both effectiveness as well as efficiency. Put simply and directly, managed care is interested in treatments that work, that do so as quickly and expeditiously as possible, and for which there is both a solid foundation of experience and ongoing proof of effect.

At a purely operational level, managed behavioral care attempts to drive treatment in directions of effective and efficient interventions and to do so, wherever possible, guided by the applicable clinical and health services research literature and relevant clinical experience. In many respects, managed care is merely putting into practice (and equally, if not more importantly, paying for) interventions that have long been known to clinicians but that have not always been reimbursable under traditional indemnity insurance plans. For example, empirical support for the effectiveness and cost savings associated with the use of alternatives to psychiatric hospitalization, such as partial hospitalization and residential, nonhospital-based treatment settings, has been building for over twenty years in the refereed scientific literature. As early as 1983, concern about the failure to translate this research support into actual practice was being openly expressed in the pages of the *New England Journal of Medicine* (Mosher, 1983). Yet it has only been with the growth and influence of managed care that these alternatives are becoming not just available but, more importantly, recognized and utilized as unique and independent parts of the continuum of care. The same is true of alternatives to program-driven inpatient treatment for substance abuse, where managed care has had a major impact on the translation of research findings into clinical practice (Giles, 1993).

It is important to point out, however, that in providing empirical support for the efficiency and effectiveness of alternatives to inpatient care, managed care is in no way broadly attacking the legitimacy of inpatient hospitalization for a wide range of clinical conditions and presentations. Instead, once again, it is seeking to maximize the clinical gains associated with the unique features of the inpatient environment (maximal control and observation of patients) by matching these features to an appropriate set of clinical indications. In general, then, managed care tends to view the inpatient setting as essential to the rapid evaluation and stabilization of certain crises but not as a necessarily essential vehicle for the traditional therapeutic work of the inpatient milieu. In fact, managed care most often looks to partial hospitalization and other structured outpatient environments for the accomplishment of those same therapeutic tasks.

Three Generations of Managed Care

If one accepts that the basic premise of managed behavioral care is to reduce variability in the treatment of mental illness and chemical dependency, it becomes clear that, over time, managed care has changed its tools and tactics. In fact, I believe that there have been at least three distinct generations of managed behavioral care, each in turn attempting to address the problems and failures of the preceding generation. Before the creation of specialty managed behavioral care organizations, some oversight of psychiatric and substance abuse care was provided by generic utilization review firms and processes. In their earliest form, they reviewed cases against empirically derived norms of length of stay for any given diagnosis. Tables existed which derived normative lengths of stay for psychiatric and chemical dependency patients, with some attempts to adjust the data for both patient and provider characteristics (Commission on Professional and Hospital Activities, 1987). The very real failure of this approach, however, was that none of the independent or case-mix variables selected, particularly diagnosis, explained much about length of stay in real life. A diagnosis such as schizophrenia, for example, associated as it is with a chronic course associated with multiple relapses and remissions, says little if anything about an individual patient's need at any given point in time for the structure and support that only an inpatient facility can provide.

In response to the shortcomings of this normative approach to oversight of psychiatric and chemical dependency care, the first generation of specialty managed care organizations developed in a number of geographic areas, in particular Minnesota and California (Bartlett, 1991). These organizations were characterized by their clinical expertise in the fields of mental health and chemical dependency treatments as well as by their attempts to make case-specific judgments about the appropriateness, efficiency, and effectiveness of proposed treatment plans. Unlike earlier attempts to apply only normative data to the review of care in these areas, these organizations developed explicit criteria which were intended to address the clinical issues related to appropriateness of care decisions, with particular attention to level-of-care determinations.

These so-called criteria were applied, usually by licensed mental health and substance abuse professionals, in the review of individual cases with providers. At their best, these reviews were characterized by creative and flexible attempts to develop individualized treatment plans for patients; at their worst, they were experienced by providers and patients alike as arbitrary and intrusive interruptions of the previously sacrosanct doctor-patient relationship. A number of the structural elements of this first generation led to its often being experienced as coercive and confrontational; these included the oft-quoted "proprietary" nature of the criteria, which remained until the early 1990s secret and unavailable to providers at large, and the fact that most providers had in no way agreed to participate in oversight of their treatment planning. These first generation programs, then, represented attempts to inspect quality and introduce uniformity into the highly variable treatment environment of the unmanaged system and to do so without any formal agreement or mutually recognized authority to do so. After all, the requirements for precertification and concurrent review were features of the insurance coverage, not decisions of the providers or the patients.

It was the seemingly coercive and confrontational nature of this first generation of managed behavioral care programs that led in the late 1980s and early 1990s to the development of a second generation. These new programs were characterized by conscious attempts on the part of the managed care organizations to promote and elicit the consent of both the patient and the provider to engage in the oversight process. This generation of consent, which is currently at its height, has been characterized by products and programs that center around so-called networks of providers who are screened to varying degrees and then selected for their general compatibility with a managed approach to treatment. After this selection process, which includes a formal review of credentials, is completed, the providers are offered formal contracts that clearly outline both the rights and responsibilities of all parties. The "consent" of consumers to have their care reviewed for medical appropriateness is elicited by promoting their use of these screened and selected providers through the availability of enhanced in-network benefits (for example, lower cost sharing and higher limits); consumers are, however, provided an opportunity to limit such review by choosing a traditional indemnity benefit for care received from noncontract providers.

This second generation has also been characterized by greater openness about and sharing of documented clinical standards. To date, a number of the larger national vendors of such services have published their criteria for making level-of-care decisions. This sharing of standards has begun to address the concern of many providers about having their treatment plans inspected against secret and sometimes vague criteria and in and of itself has helped to reduce the variability of treatment approaches reflected in the practice patterns of many providers.

In fact, this aspect of cooperation and even collaboration between provider and managed care organization is at the heart of the next generation of managed care. This third generation involves the development of organized delivery systems in mental health and substance abuse that center around value-added relationships between providers with demonstrated and documented managed care compatibility and their associated managed care partners (Freeman, 1992). Such features as reduction or even elimination of case-level management, expedited claim payment, and transfer of financial risk and clinical accountability are routinely being explored and implemented by the more sophisticated managed care vendors nationally. Under these programs, oversight moves from the level of the individual case to the level of practice patterns. Moreover, increasingly it involves not just the quantitative review of utilization and financial data but also examination of the direct clinical and indirect nonclinical effects of the treatments provided. By building into such organized systems the routine and methodologically sound evaluation of information about a wide variety of treatment outcomes, and, more importantly, by applying this data to validate or identify shortcomings in clinical standards and treatment approaches, the infrastructure for truly accountable, improvable delivery of mental health and chemical dependency services is being developed (Bartlett, 1993).

Controversy over Quality

This latest and still developing generation of managed behavioral care programs provides both the opportunity and the vehicle to address the single greatest controversy that has surrounded the field since its inception, that of quality. In its attempts to reduce the wide variability of treatment approaches that have prevailed in the delivery of mental health and substance abuse treatments, managed care has continually opened itself to charges of delivering care that was of poorer quality than that available in the unmanaged fee-for-service sector. To date, the response that managed care attempts to base its choices wherever possible on the available clinical and health services research literature, as was discussed earlier, has not proved adequate to quiet these concerns. And this is perhaps understandable in the light of the fact that the available literature, although powerful in places, is both too general and too incomplete to address the clinical realities of all patients.

The key point to take away from this situation, however, is not that limiting variability in and of itself contributes to any decline in quality of care. In fact, I maintain that managed care seeks to reduce variability in treatment approach in order to drive quality, not reduce it. The quality of which I speak, however, is not a subjective, ill-defined quality known only to a small group of insiders, but rather an objective, measurable, and ultimately improvable type of quality. In this regard, the approach of managed care is being shaped by the significant changes currently underway in many areas of U.S. business in the definition and management of quality. This "quality revolution" goes under many names, such as continuous quality improvement and Total Quality Management, but whatever the name, its goal is the measurement and the demonstrable improvement of quality over time, and its prophets are W. Edwards Deming, J. M. Juran, and Philip B. Crosby. The process is one of defining objective standards of quality and managing the variation around these standards; the result is not mindless uniformity, it is reduction of waste, rework, and unneeded complexity.

It becomes easy, then, to differentiate this approach to quality from that which has traditionally held sway in health care, namely the review of individual cases against subjective criteria. Under this approach, quality was defined and bestowed much as in any guild. Now, however, the paradigm for determining and measuring quality in health care is changing from that of the craftsperson to that of the engineer, and a core component of this change is the requirement for objective, documented standards of care. What the third generation of managed care organizations will be able to do is to apply these standards of care in the context of delivery systems designed to continuously evaluate the results of the application. Many managed behavioral care organizations are developing and even deploying the capability of tracking a variety of outcomes of care, both clinical (for example, symptom reduction or functional status) and nonclinical (for example, satisfaction with care or quality of life) on an ongoing and cost-effective basis. This capability, in turn, provides the foundation for the ongoing empirical investigation of what truly constitutes cost-effective and efficient care. Moreover, it will also provide the ability to continually evaluate and improve approaches to treatment as new and different ones become available.

Conclusion

In what would be perhaps the ultimate irony, managed care may well become a major vehicle through which defensible and demonstrable standards of care are developed and refined. More importantly, what was originally perceived as an assault on the practice of the behavioral health care professions may well be a major force in the demonstration of their value and, in doing so, may well be instrumental in the efforts to preserve and, we hope, even expand access to appropriate and affordable care in mental health and substance abuse areas.

References

Bartlett, J. "The Growth of Networks in Mental Health and Substance Abuse Care: The Recent California Experience." *Journal of Ambulatory Care Management,* 1991, *14* (4), 18–26.

Bartlett, J. "Behavioral Healthcare Tomorrow—Evolution or Revolution?" *Behavioral Healthcare Tomorrow,* 1993, *1,* 30–34.

Commission on Professional and Hospital Activities. *Psychiatric Length of Stay.* Ann Arbor, Mich.: CPHA Publications, 1987.

Eisenberg, L. "Treating Depression & Anxiety in Primary Care." *New England Journal of Medicine,* 1992, *326* (16), 1080–1084.

Freeman, M. "Perspectives on the Future of Network-Based Managed Behavioral Care Systems." *American Association of Preferred Provider Organizations Journal,* 1992, 2 (2), 36–40.

Garfield, S. L. "Research on Client Variables in Psychotherapy." In S. L. Garfield and A. E. Bergin (eds.), *Handbook of Psychotherapy and Behavior Change.* New York: Wiley, 1986.

Giles, T. "Managed Mental Health Care and Effective Psychotherapy." *Journal of Behavioral Therapy and Experimental Psychiatry,* 1991, *22,* 83–86.

Giles, T. *Managed Mental Health Care: A Guide for Practitioners, Employers, and Hospital Administrators.* Boston: Allyn & Bacon, 1993.

J. Foster Higgins. *1992 Health Care Benefits Survey.* Cleveland, Ohio: J. Foster Higgins, 1992.

Mosher, L. "Alternatives to Psychiatric Hospitalization." *New England Journal of Medicine,* 1983, *309* (25), 1579–1580.

Myers, J. K., Weissman, M. M., Tischler, G. L., Holzer, C. E., Leaf, P. J., Orvaschel, H., Anthony, J. C., Boyd, J. H., Burke, J. D., Kramer, M., and Stolzman, R. "Six-Month Prevalence of Psychiatric Disorders in Three Communities." *Archives of General Psychiatry,* 1984, *41,* 959–967.

National Association of Psychiatric Health Systems. *1993 Survey Report on Utilization Management Firms Conducting Psychiatric Review.* Washington, D.C.: National Association of Psychiatric Health Systems, 1993.

JOHN BARTLETT, M.D., M.P.H., is vice president/corporate medical director of MCC Behavioral Care, Inc., in Eden Prairie, Minnesota.

As psychiatric management of the mentally ill shifts away from prolonged and continuous inpatient hospitalization toward a surgical model of care, knowledge and skill in short-term symptom suppression and stabilization, psychoeducation, collaboration with the family, and posthospital planning are essential to success.

Unbundling the Function of an Inpatient Unit

Ira D. Glick

This chapter will describe the primary function of inpatient psychiatric units in the new era of managed care. Over the past two decades, psychiatric management of both the acutely and chronically mentally ill has shifted away from prolonged and continuous inpatient hospitalization toward repeated brief hospitalizations. The locus has changed from large public hospitals to various outpatient settings. In the 1950s, the psychiatric hospitals were at the center of a wheel of services and referrals originating from outpatient settings, families, and, not uncommonly, the police. In the 1990s, outpatient services are at the center of the wheel, and referrals to those services come not only from the psychiatric hospitals but also from loci that previously had referred nearly exclusively to those hospitals. For some patients, this shift has resulted in frequent readmissions, or in a low level of psychosocial functioning, for those in the community, and in a marked increase in homelessness.

In the United States, the shortening of hospital stays has been related to three factors. The first factor is economic, that is, cost containment and cost shifting from state to federal governments. The second is ideologic and concerns the pursuit of the "least restrictive environment," that is, the desire to treat the patient in the setting in which there is maximum "freedom." The third is political, that is, government money has been shifted away from inpatient services. Unfortunately, these changes have mostly occurred *not* as a result of

Sections of this chapter are reprinted from I. D. Glick, N. Y. Freund, and M. Olfson, "What a Psychiatric Hospitalization Can and Cannot Do: A Review of Efficacy Studies," in E. Persad, S. S. Kazarian, and L. W. Joseph (eds.), *The Mental Hospital in the 21st Century* (Toronto: Wall & Emerson, 1992), pp. 191–204, by permission of the publisher.

new scientific information (with certain exceptions in the controlled studies that I will discuss later).

Concurrently with the shift toward outpatient treatment and brief hospitalizations (largely in community hospitals), the population being served within the psychiatric hospital is being experienced as more difficult to treat. The increased occurrence of dual diagnosis—violent symptoms and concurrent medical illness—among the remaining hospital population contributes to these individuals' being difficult to treat. An important question is, Why has the hospitalized population changed? In the United States, part of the answer certainly lies in the skimming of patients with better prognoses to private and for-profit psychiatric hospitals and in the more restrictive admissions policies at other inpatient facilities. In addition, a frequent perception of inpatient staffs is that the families (in the broadest sense) of these patients are less available—that is, less willing to be involved with treatment—and possess less financial and social resources than formerly.

Finally, over the last two decades there have been some major advances in diagnoses and therapy that have important implications for hospital treatment. The first is a more reliable and valid diagnostic system, for example, DSM-III and DSM-III-R. The second is new medications such as clozapine and new uses for older medications (for example, Tegretol for lithium refractory bipolar disorder). And, finally, there are new family intervention strategies based on findings demonstrating a decrease in the rate of relapse when family intervention is prescribed.

We are currently being called upon to redefine the function of the inpatient hospital in the context of all these changes. Drawing on the lessons learned from past research on the efficacy of inpatient psychiatry, a better understanding of the populations we will be treating, and technological advances in treatment capabilities, the remainder of the chapter gives a brief account of an appropriate new role for inpatient psychiatry.

Controlled Studies Review

In the 1970s, there were six major controlled studies comparing long-term to short-term hospitalization. Table 3.1 details each of these studies. A careful examination of this table reveals that in almost every study, except that by Glick and Hargreaves, shorter-term was as efficacious as longer-term hospitalization. In addition, it was shown that longer hospitalization tended to behaviorally condition the patient and the family to seek hospitalization during times of stress. The study carried out by Glick and Hargreaves (1979) suggested that certain patients, those with acute schizophrenia and affective disorder, might benefit from a longer-term hospitalization. Glick and Hargreaves believed the reason might be that the longer hospitalization allowed the patient and the family to learn something about the illness and begin to make workable plans for aftercare. Certainly, in the presence of adequate aftercare services, the shorter-term hospitalization seemed to be the treatment of choice for most patients.

In 1980, Test and Stein published findings from their important project examining community-based intensive treatment versus short-term standard hospitalization plus standard aftercare (Test and Stein; Weisbrod, Test, and Stein). Their results showed that the experimental group of patients was hospitalized for fewer days and demonstrated improved social and occupational functioning and reduced clinical symptoms. But when the project stopped, the results washed out. An important (and obvious) lesson from this and other community treatment studies is that severely ill psychiatric patients require *continuous* treatment. It is also important to emphasize that we still know very little about what actually occurs during a hospitalization and how the treat-

Table 3.1. Long-Term Versus Short-Term Hospitalization

Research Group	*Design (All Random Assignments)*	*Design Problems*	*Outcome After Follow-Up Period*
Caffey, Galbrecht, and Klett (1971)	Short (21 days) vs. standard (80 days), with aftercare controlled	Groups overlap, no drug controls, males, chronic VA patients.	Long-term treatment offered no advantage over short-term treatment for schizophrenia.
Glick and Hargreaves (1979)	Short-term (21-28 days) vs. long-term (90-120 days)	Aftercare confounded.	Long-term offered significant advantages over short-term for good prehospital functioning schizophrenics, especially females, and possibly for patients with affective disorder. Long-term offered no advantage over short-term for patients with personality disorder and for schizophrenic patients with a history of poor prehospital functioning.
Herz, Endicott, and Spitzer (1977)	Very short (11 days) with day hospital vs. very short without day hospital vs. long-term (60 days)	Patients with families only.	Long-term not only offered no advantage over a combination of very short hospitalization plus day hospital, but in fact, very short term patients functioned better, had less psychopathology and were considered less of a burden on the family at one-year follow-up.
Rosen, Mattes, and Klein (1977)	Long-term (90 days) vs. standard very long (average 180 days)	Aftercare confounded, not strictly random assignment.	Very long term offered no advantages over long-term when all diagnoses were combined or when schizophrenia or personality disorder was examined separately. Group therapy had a significant positive outcome.
Hirsch, Platt, and Knights (1979)	Brief (9 days) vs. standard (17 days)	Aftercare confounded.	Few differences between groups at one-year follow-up, including no difference in burden.
Kennedy and Hird (1980)	Brief (11 days) vs. standard (24 days)	Aftercare confounded, patients excluded for whom continuity of care was an issue.	No significant difference between groups on rehospitalization or psychopathology, but standard group patients had significantly more contact with their general practitioners.

Source: Glick, Freund, and Olson, 1992. Reprinted by permission.

ments provided bring about recovery. Given limited resources, this is a crucial area for future study.

Clinical Implications

The message from the data in these controlled studies can be summarized as follows:

Outpatient treatment is more advantageous than inpatient.
Short-term hospitalization is more advantageous than long-term (if outpatient services available).
Short-term hospitalization is indicated for most patients with schizophrenia, especially *females.*
Long-term hospitalization is indicated for schizophrenia with *good* prehospital functioning.
Short-term hospitalization is indicated for schizophrenia with *poor* prehospital functioning (the patients will seek or stay in treatment posthospital).
Patients with three- to sixty-day hospitalization do no worse than patients with longer hospitalization with respect to global outcome, symptoms, social and vocational functioning, or risk of rehospitalization over eighteen to twenty-four months.

It is important to note that the fourth and fifth implications are exactly the opposite of some conventional wisdom. I explain this as follows: patients with good prognosis can benefit in the long run from the extra time in the hospital. On the other hand, patients with chronic poor functioning are better served by hospital management of relapses with the bulk of their ongoing treatment occurring on an outpatient basis, since they are not able to use the resources of the hospital when acutely ill.

The literature reviewed here leads me to suggest a "new" and somewhat controversial model of hospitalization. This model, of course, represents an idealized version—a hope for the future, rather than a current reality. I propose that, to best serve the vast majority of mentally ill patients now requiring admission, the psychiatric hospital should become more like an acute medical service, or a surgical suite, than an asylum. The psychiatric staff must be more like a surgical or medical team. I believe the objectives are the same as for medical hospitalizations, that is, most patients with chronic coronary disease or respiratory disease come in for stabilization or for a new posthospital treatment plan. The usual reasons for hospitalization relate to the natural history of the illness (for example, narrowing of the coronary arteries or medication noncompliance). Therefore, the new model is similar to a surgeon's removing a tumor or an internist's treating a diabetic in ketoacidosis. The surgeon will ultimately refer his patient for radiation therapy or chemotherapy and will see the patient frequently to evaluate him or her for recurrence. The internist will manage the metabolic emergency, assess what caused the decompensation, and then adjust the patient's insulin, diet, and general outpatient management.

Thus, at the time of each admission, the psychiatric hospital team of the twenty-first century will have a problem-oriented focus which will be directed at well-defined tasks that can be done only in the hospital. It will involve a major intervention for *both* patient and family and will result in considerable distress to *both* before things improve. It will be like an operation in which a lot of blood is spilled, but subsequently, things get better. In addition, the psychiatric hospital of the twenty-first century will do what other medical services are now doing to an increasing degree, that is, educate patients about their illness and its treatment. An example occurs in the field of obstetrics when pregnant patients and their spouses are prepared for labor and delivery with Lamaze classes. The patients are given extensive instruction on everything they need to know about infants, from breast feeding and normal growth and development to bathing and diapering.

Objectives inherent in the surgical model of psychiatric hospitalization include short-term symptom suppression and stabilization, psychoeducation of the patient and family, collaboration with the family, and induction into posthospital treatment for both patient and family. The central issue is to set objectives appropriate to the needs of each patient and to the optimal length of stay for each disorder. Of course, there is by definition a need for adequate security and cost-efficient staffing, based on patient census, rapidity of turnover, and illness; and finally, and most importantly, effective communication systems to allow for a true integration of treatment and an efficient treatment process.

The main components of this model and key means of obtaining these goals will be discussed in turn.

Short-Term Symptom Suppression and Stabilization. The diagnosis will be "quick and dirty." We do not have the luxury of a three- to four-week patient workup. Working diagnoses have to be made in the first twenty-four to forty-eight hours. Prehospital screening can do much to eliminate useless and ineffective hospitalizations. Knowing where one is headed before one gets started greatly increases the chances of reaching one's destination. To do this screening, key historical information, collected prior to hospitalization from relatives, other hospitals, and therapists, is crucial. Needless to say, we need to develop techniques to obtain this information, including use of computer data banks.

Treatment goals must be clinically reasonable and attainable within the existing constraints. The goals should be more modest than they have previously been. A major goal will be to reduce the probability of posthospital relapse. By necessity, the decision to discharge will have to be based on options for aftercare and the nature of the illness.

Treatment should consist of sequential treatment trials. Accordingly, plans for these trials should be made very soon (presumably the first day) after admission—for example, a trial of medication A; if that does not work, medication B; if that does not work, medications C plus D. Once patients are in the trial mode, the trials can be started in the hospital but continued following discharge. It needs to be emphasized that these somatic therapies must be given in adequate amounts. Psychotherapy is also of use but must be modified, given the cognitive impairments that are so common in severely ill psychiatric patients.

Psychoeducation. The 1990s, I think, may be the age of psychoeducation, as a number of studies have now found that psychoeducation is associated with better outcome (Greenberg and others, 1980; Anderson, Hogarty, and Reiss, 1980). We have also seen in the eighties the flowering of the consumer movement on behalf of the mentally ill. Such organizations as (National Alliance for Research on Schizophrenia and Depression (NARSAD), the National Mental Health Association, the National Alliance for the Mentally Ill, the Manic Depressive Disease Association, and others have all been important forces in the improvement of treatment for the mentally ill.

Family Collaboration. In my view, hospitalization without family (or significant others) or case managers involved in treatment stands little chance of success in the long run. The role of the patient and his or her support system in treatment is crucial. Likewise, the staff must do everything possible to enlist the patient's active participation in the treatment process regardless of the patient's initial presentation. The focus should be on involving the family in the appropriate treatments. The family will be viewed as able to become expert in some of the techniques to help manage their ill member. The treatment team helps with other options.

Posthospital Planning. Given the components just described, a strong push must be made to involve the patient, the family, and the referring professionals as part of the treatment team in order to develop a posthospital plan. This work should start prior to admission and must continue through the hospitalization and posthospital phase. Facilitating prompt posthospital placement of patients means determining the aftercare plans early as well as speeding up testing. For example, psychological testing that arrives on the day of discharge is of little use. Other important strategies include monitoring blood levels, using electroconvulsive therapy (ECT) when appropriate, and using a seven-day hospital schedule. These efforts should improve the treatment efficiency of the hospital.

In order to successfully implement these goals, the introduction of the techniques suggested above is warranted. These techniques are summarized in the following list:

Prehospital *screening* to plan hospital objectives
Prehospital obtaining of *information* from relatives and therapists
Prehospital agreement of *significant others* to participate in hospitalization
Greater use of *medical model* techniques with less reliance on *milieu model* techniques
Sequential trials
Combination therapy
Greater use of *somatic* therapies (adequate amount and duration versus risks)
Greater use of *family* intervention and lesser use of *individual* and group therapy (with increased use of educational strategies)

Introduction of *individual psychoeducation*
Introduction of *family psychoeducation*
Introduction of increased *efficiency:* speed up lab and psychological tests, monitor blood levels, adopt seven-day schedule, minimize one-to-one intensive nursing.

The following list outlines factors that enable the hospitalization to be more effective. Of course, these are ideals not usually fully achieved in practice.

A detailed history of past treatments and the patient's response to these interventions
A willing patient who is able to comply with treatment
A history of positive response to the planned treatment, or data indicating that the treatment planned during the inpatient stay is efficacious for that particular problem
The presence of a social support group willing and able to be involved in hospital and posthospital treatment.

Next we look at the absolute and relative indications for hospitalization. The relative indications usually (but not always) involve hospitalization; for example, treatments like ECT can sometimes can be given in the community.

Absolute Indications
A need to provide safety and security for patients for whom:
 Symptoms are so disturbing, to the patient or society, that the patient cannot be managed outside the hospital
 Overt and serious homicidal or suicidal ideation is present (including acute exacerbation of chronic symptoms)
A need to provide crisis stabilization treatment of special populations; for example, geriatric psychiatry, medically ill psychiatric patients, substance abusers, and so forth.

Relative Indications
A need to change or initiate a sequential medication or ECT trial, that is, aggressive somatic management
A need to carry out a treatment that almost always has to be done in a hospital (for example, ECT)
A need to observe the patient in a controlled setting in order to clarify diagnosis or to change drug management, that is, intensive evaluation
A need to manage the chronic patient whose deficits have led to intrapsychic or interpersonal problems resulting in noncompliance or decompensation.

Finally, the following items describe a number of situations in which hospitalization may be contraindicated:

Repeating a previously failed treatment for the same reasons it was tried before (such as rehospitalizing a patient who recurrently cuts his or her wrists, without offering any new treatment interventions)

Trying a host of treatments in the hope that "something will work"

Attempting to bring about major character changes or alterations in family structure (although such treatment may be initiated during a short hospitalization)

Washing out all drug effects and starting medication anew when the patient's history indicates a likelihood of poor response to the new medication

Trying to convince the patient and the family to change a living situation when both have no desire to do so

Sheltering malingerers or patients facing legal charges who enter the hospital to avoid a court date, or providing shelter to the homeless

Using the hospital to accomplish a task (such as making minor medication adjustments) that could be accomplished as efficaciously in an outpatient setting.

Unanswered Questions

I am indebted to Cournos (1987), who has pointed out some of the limitations of current models of hospitalization. Some patients are severely ill, do not respond to medication, or do not improve enough to leave the hospital. They remain an unanswered challenge to the profession and probably asylum is needed for them. Cournos also points out that some patients improve but do not sustain the gains after the hospitalization. For them, one possibility is day hospitals. Hospitalization for adolescents also remains a major issue. Although long-term hospitalization is heavily used in North America for the treatment of disturbed adolescents, there are no data indicating greater efficacy with hospitalization compared to outpatient treatment. The increase in the current population of patients being hospitalized with associated substance abuse, the so-called dual diagnosis patients, as well as inpatients with associated medical problems and patients with violent behaviors, presents a special challenge to the hospitals. At present, specialized treatments are lacking for these important patient groups.

More study is needed of alternative residential placements and of different kinds of staffing strategies for different diagnostic groups. In addition, studies of longer-term hospitalization also need to be done. The questions here are, For whom is hospitalization indicated? and, Who will pay?

Conclusion

I have reviewed changes in delivery of mental health services, outlined objectives of psychiatric hospitalization, and described the controlled literature pertaining to the efficacy of psychiatric hospitalization. I suggest that the psychiatric hospital of the twenty-first century will be more like an acute medical and surgical service than like its historical roles as prison, asylum, rest home, or long-stay facility. That is, given the short-term nature of most hospitalizations, the aims are to make accurate psychiatric and medical diagnoses, begin symptom stabilization, provide psychoeducation, rework posthospital plans, initiate treatment, and consult with outpatient clinicians, the patient, and the family.

All of us look forward to the day when we, as professionals can provide the data to make the hospital a safe, helpful, cost-efficient, and more humane environment for the improved treatment of our patients and their families.

References

Anderson, C., Hogarty, G. E., and Reiss, D. J. "Family Treatment of Adult Schizophrenic Patients: A Psychoeducational Approach." *Schizophrenia Bulletin,* 1980, *6,* 490–505.

Cournos, F. "Hospitalization Outcome Studies: Implications for the Treatment of the Very Ill Patient." *Psychiatric Clinics of North America,* 1987, *10,* 165–176.

Glick, I. D., Freund, N. Y., and Olfson, M. "What a Psychiatric Hospitalization Can and Cannot Do: A Review of Efficacy Studies." In E. Persad, S. S. Kazarian, and L. W. Joseph (eds.), *The Mental Hospital in the 21st Century* (pp. 191–204). Toronto: Wall & Emerson, 1992.

Glick, I. D., and Hargreaves, W. A. *Psychiatric Hospital Treatment for the 1980s: A Controlled Study of Short Versus Long Hospitalization.* Lexington, Mass.: Lexington Press, 1979.

Greenberg, L., Fine, S. B., Cohen, C., Larson, K., Michaelson, A., Rubinton, P., and Glick, I. D. "An Interdisciplinary Psychoeducation Program for Schizophrenic Patients and Their Families in an Acute Care Setting." *Hospital & Community Psychiatry,* 1980, *39,* 277–282.

Test, M. A., and Stein, L. I. "Alternative to Mental Hospital Treatment: Social Costs." *Archives of General Psychiatry,* 1980, *37,* 409–411.

Weisbrod, B. A., Test, M. A., and Stein, L. I. "Alternative to Mental Hospital Treatment: Economic Benefit-Cost Analysis." *Archives of General Psychiatry,* 1980, *37,* 400–405.

IRA D. GLICK, M.D., is professor of psychiatry at Stanford University School of Medicine.

Part Two

Treatment of Specific Clinical Populations

Pressure for briefer hospitalizations creates greater challenges in treating dual diagnosis patients, making it important to understand the scope of the problem, the relationships between psychiatric disorders and chemical dependence, brief assessment and intervention approaches, and relapse prevention methods.

Brief Inpatient Treatment of Dual Diagnosis Patients

Emil Chiauzzi

In recent years clinicians working with both addictive and psychiatric disorders have become aware of the overlap between these populations. Those working in psychiatric settings note the obstacles to gaining an accurate assessment of psychiatric symptoms in the presence of addictive substances. Similarly, those working in addictions settings often find that chronically relapsing patients are experiencing underlying psychiatric problems. The concurrence between chemical dependence and psychiatric disorders is noteworthy.

Scope of the Dual Diagnosis Problem

Kosten and Kleber (1988) report that as many as 30 to 50 percent of psychiatric patients and 80 percent of addicted patients can be categorized as dually diagnosed. The overlap between affective disorders and depressant substance use is quite dramatic. Forty percent of patients seeking treatment for alcoholism met criteria for an affective disorder, while 30 to 40 percent of those presenting with affective disorders were abusing alcohol or other depressant drugs (Weiss and Rosenberg, 1985). About 10 to 30 percent of alcoholics experience panic disorder and 20 percent of anxiety disordered patients abuse alcohol (Cox, Norton, Swinson, and Endler, 1990). Ross, Glaser, and Germanson (1988) report that about two-thirds of alcoholics initiating treatment have symptoms that resemble anxiety disorders. The lifetime prevalence of schizophrenics who experience substance abuse disorders is between 10 and 65 percent (Mueser, Bellack, and Blanchard, 1992). The risk of schizophrenia in alcoholics is about four times as high as in nonalcoholics (Helzer and Pryzbeck, 1988). The presence of psychiatric disorders in cocaine addicts is also significant, with high prevalence rates of depression, bipolar disorder, and attention deficit disorder (Group for the Advancement of Psychiatry Committee on Alcoholism and the Addictions, 1991). As many as 75 percent of opiate addicts experience major depression (Rounsaville, Weissman, Kleber, and Wilber, 1982).

The term *dual diagnosis* usually refers to Axis I disorders, but many addicted individuals meet criteria for personality disorders. One survey of inpatient substance abuse patients found that 57 percent had Axis II disorders (Nace, Davis, and Gaspari, 1991). These patients used more illegal drugs, reported less satisfaction with their lives, and evidenced greater impulsivity than those substance abusers without personality disorders. The most common Axis II diagnosis is antisocial personality disorder, with rates among alcoholic men ranging up to 50 percent and alcoholic women ranging up to 20 percent (Blume, 1989). Borderline personality disorders were second highest in frequency, occurring in about 10 to 20 percent of cases (Mirin and Weiss, 1991). Addicted individuals with borderline personality disorders are particularly relapse-prone, as they manifest poorer impulse control, impaired reality testing, greater dysphoria, and more antisocial behavior than those without borderline pathology.

The combination of psychiatric and addictive disorders is associated with significant impairment and poorer treatment outcome. The best predictor of relapse in addictions is psychiatric severity, that is, addicted patients with severe psychiatric disorders have difficulty benefiting from inpatient and/or outpatient addiction treatments (McLellan and others, 1983). Conversely, those with low psychiatric severity can benefit from virtually any type of addiction treatment.

The combination of psychiatric disorders and chemical dependence is quite disruptive to the treatment process, as these patients evidence greater aggressiveness, hostility, and noncompliance with treatment (Drake, McLaughlin, Pepper, and Minkoff, 1991). These tendencies interfere with development of the coping skills necessary to managing practical aspects of daily living, such as maintaining residential stability, and increase the likelihood of patient relapse and institutionalization in hospitals and jails.

Relationships Between Psychiatric Disorders and Chemical Dependence

What are the relationships between psychiatric disorders and chemical dependence? Psychopathology and addiction may coexist in several ways: Axis I or II disorders may increase the risk of addiction; the course of addiction may be altered by psychiatric symptoms; the course of psychopathology may be altered by substance use; addiction may create psychopathology, which may then persist after substance abuse is discontinued; and psychopathology and addiction may originate from a common vulnerability (Meyer, 1986). The complexity of these relationships renders rigid clinical conceptualizations (for example, that the psychiatric disorder is *always* primary) hazardous and may actually produce poorer outcomes. Individual assessment among dual diagnosis individuals is paramount and should account for differential effects of substances among disorders, changes in psychiatric status as a result of substance use, and perceived psychological benefits in using substances.

Linkages between psychopathology and addiction may vary from disorder to disorder. For example, affective disorders and substance abuse do not simply coexist but each affects the course of the other. Affective disorders increase the risk of substance abuse, and these disorders also share common vulnerabilities (Bukstein, Brent, and Kaminer, 1989). Depression may reduce treatment compliance, while alcohol use may reduce the efficacy of depression treatment. Alcoholics with depression generally begin drinking at an earlier age and progress to problem drinking sooner than alcoholics without additional psychopathology. Familial affective disorders may also serve as risk factors for substance abuse. It should also be noted that "alcohol abuse is often the 'horse' to the 'cart' of major depressive disorder" (Vaillant, 1993, p. 95).

The relationships between anxiety and substance abuse also vary (Bukstein, Brent, and Kaminer, 1989). There is a high concurrence of agoraphobia, phobias, and panic disorders with substance abuse. These conditions may result from symptoms of withdrawal from alcohol, opiates, or barbiturates; self-medication of tension; or a family history of anxiety disorders among alcoholics. About 25 percent of these patients develop an anxiety disorder *after* a period of substance abuse (Mirin and Weiss, 1991).

Schizophrenics may utilize substances to reduce symptoms such as poverty of speech, affective flattening, anhedonia, asociality, attention impairment, or dysphoria (Schneier and Siris, 1987). However, schizophrenics who use alcohol may further compromise cognitive functions such as memory. Mueser, Bellack, and Blanchard (1992) report that alcohol use has been associated with higher vulnerability to relapses and that stimulant use can precipitate an earlier onset of schizophrenia in high-risk individuals.

Brief Assessment and Intervention Guidelines

Because of the limited time available in inpatient treatment, it is critical for clinicians to be aware of stages of change as they apply to both addictions and psychiatric disorders.

Stages of Change. DiClemente (1991), describing the work of James Prochaska, delineates therapeutic change in addictive and psychiatric disorders into five phases: precontemplation, which comprises the "four R's of reluctance, rebellion, resignation, and rationalization; contemplation, during which the patient recognizes the need for change but remains ambivalent; determination, which involves a decision to change; action, during which a plan is implemented and appropriate recovery and coping skills are learned; and maintenance, which requires the continuation of newly learned skills through relapse prevention. Most psychotherapies devote maximum effort to implementation of change strategies, but the high incidence of relapse suggests the need for greater attention to maintenance. Many people "recycle" and can revert even to a precontemplative stance. As a result, clinical activity should confront the obstacles to "staying stopped" even more than the initial cessation of addictive and psychiatric symptoms.

Dual diagnosis patients may present at several different phases of change during the course of short-term inpatient treatment. For those in the precontemplation phase, the clinician should seek to increase cognitive dissonance by providing objective information that conflicts with the patient's perceptions of his symptoms. Objective, data-oriented assessments, such as psychological testing, laboratory results, and empirical information about dual diagnosis issues, may yield better results. The patient who is already contemplating change may still be quite ambivalent, so the primary goal should be to emphasize the negative consequences of the addiction; provide education about the rewards of recovery; remove obstacles to change (for example, explain the likely progression of withdrawal); and increase a sense of mastery of coping skills (for example, through providing contact with successful recovering people who can model appropriate behavior). During the determination phase, the task of the clinician revolves around specification of a treatment contract. Typical provisions would be explanation of a method of detoxification; specification of amount and type of educational, psychotherapeutic, psychiatric, and self-help interventions; family therapy, as a means of collecting clinical data and educating significant others; compliance with a psychotropic medications regimen; and agreement to avoid substitute addictive substances or behaviors. The final two phases will be discussed later in this chapter.

Brief Assessment Principles. There are five areas that are critical in the short-term assessment of dual diagnosis patients: the patient's denial of either the psychiatric condition or the addiction; the overlap between psychiatric and withdrawal symptoms; the importance of historical data; the utility of objective *measures* of symptoms and progress; and the utility of patients' subjective impressions of their dual disorders.

Address denial. Denial is usually associated with addiction but can also occur with psychiatric disorders. It is especially evident in dual diagnosis patients, as one disorder can fuel denial of the other. For example, an anxious patient addicted to alprazolam may blame his physician for prescribing benzodiazepines. An addicted patient may regard severe depression simply as a consequence of alcoholism, with the expectation that abstinence will eliminate depressive symptoms. Past treatment settings are also important. Dual diagnosis patients who have been treated on chemical dependence units may accept an addiction diagnosis but deny a psychiatric diagnosis. The opposite may be true for the dual diagnosis patient treated on psychiatric units. Those who identify with the addiction may resist psychiatric formulations due to fear of appearing "crazy." Those who identify with psychiatric disorders may believe that they require alcohol or drugs to feel "normal."

In fact, substance use can interfere with progress in treatment, as the patient's ability to comply with a medication regimen or to engage in psychotherapy or treatment planning may be seriously impaired. The patient enters a revolving door of symptoms, as addictive behavior may trigger psychiatric symptoms which then may increase a tendency toward self-medication. In a brief inpatient treatment, it is critical to orient the patient regarding the parallel nature of dual disorders (Minkoff, 1991). Assessment of past relapses or past symptoms during abstinent periods can educate the patient to maintain a vigilance toward both sets of symptoms. An ignorance of either the addictive or psychiatric disorder should be construed as the beginning of the relapse process.

Differentiate withdrawal symptoms from psychiatric symptoms. This principle involves the similarities between psychiatric symptoms and withdrawal symptoms. Acute withdrawal syndromes are characterized by significant effects on physical status, cognitive functioning, and emotional presentation. Withdrawal from alcohol and benzodiazepines may give rise to irritability, tremulousness, anxiety, and even delirium. Opioid withdrawal is not life threatening but is characterized by irritability and desperation. Cocaine withdrawal often leads to a "crash," which is experienced as depression, fatigue, hypersomnia, and craving the drug for immediate relief. Marijuana withdrawal is characterized by irritability, anxiety, insomnia, and loss of appetite. Such acute symptoms should decrease within a matter of days.

In addition, psychiatric symptoms and protracted withdrawal symptoms frequently overlap. Protracted withdrawal is characterized by neuropsychological dysfunctions such as abstract reasoning problems, poor problem solving, impaired short-term memory, and visual-spatial deficits (McCrady and Smith, 1986). A high proportion of those in their first six months of abstinence report poor memory, thought blocking, trouble concentrating, or unpleasant thoughts (De Soto, O'Donnell, Allred, and Lopes, 1985). Many recovering people also experience insomnia, fatigue, distractibility, mood lability, and irritability. Approximately 75 percent of alcoholics evidence varying degrees of such cognitive dysfunction (Tarter, Ott, and Mezzich, 1991), although researchers have identified a natural course of recovery of cognitive functioning. Long-term memory functions, such as vocabulary, are generally intact throughout recovery, while verbal learning improves after two to three weeks of abstinence and short-term memory improves after one to two months of abstinence (McCrady and Smith, 1986). The ability to comprehend abstract information, including many concepts used by Alcoholics Anonymous (for example, "letting go" and "higher power") may be impaired for months or even years. The effect of protracted withdrawal on assessment is significant, as most of the above mentioned symptoms are also found in affective, anxiety, and even psychotic disorders.

Use historical data. The importance of historical data is that it can clarify the relative contributions of substance addiction and underlying psychiatric disturbances to impaired cognitive and emotional functioning. Assessment should include a review of the patient's family history of psychiatric disorders, any manifestation of psychiatric symptoms prior to the initiation of substance use, past withdrawal experiences, the duration of symptoms during past abstinent periods, and past responses to psychiatric medication.

Use objective measures. This principle suggests that even in a brief inpatient stay, formal assessment instruments can be utilized to track therapeutic response and the need for medication. For example, depression is very commonly related to withdrawal. It can be tracked with the Beck Depression Inventory and should begin to dissipate within days. Any *worsening* of Beck scores should indicate the potential for an affective disorder. However, antidepressant medication should not be prescribed unless the patient has already achieved four weeks of abstinence (Evans and Sullivan, 1990; Brown and Schuckit, 1988) or has a known psychiatric history. When the presence of a psychiatric disorder has not been established, it is prudent to wait until the symptoms stop getting better before considering a medication strategy. The use of objective measures has an added benefit—patients can be brought actively into the assessment process and encouraged to monitor objective symptoms.

Use patients' perceptions. This principle underscores the importance of experiential information in the assessment of dual disorders. Most dual diagnosis patients, by virtue of their past treatment experience and intervention, have their own perceptions of causality and the relationship between psychiatric and addictive symptoms. Regardless of the actual relationship, such patient theories can exert a powerful effect over the patient's compliance with and understanding of treatment. The patient should be given an opportunity to comment on whether early cognitive or emotional symptoms are differentially linked to psychiatric or addictive disturbance. Not only does the clinician gather information about the withdrawal process but he or she also gains an understanding about the patient's denial, insight, and/or initiative in becoming an active participant in treatment.

Brief Treatment Guidelines. The current literature on short-term treatment of dual diagnosis patients demonstrates several major principles: compliance should be operationally defined; the focus should be on low-demand, supportive treatment; multidisciplinary intervention is necessary to fully address the dual diagnosis patient's complex problems; and self-help groups should be utilized in a flexible manner.

Compliance. This term is deceptive, because it is thought to refer to simple adherence of the patient to therapeutic guidelines. However, compliance (or *motivation,* another commonly used term), likely resides within the *interaction* between clinician and patient. Miller (1985, pp. 87–88) states that "a client tends to be judged as motivated if he or she accepts the therapist's view of the problem (including the need for help and the diagnosis), is distressed, and complies with treatment prescriptions. The issue of motivation is intensified with dual diagnosis patients, who are often ambivalent and conflicted."

Many clinicians regard motivation as a trait, but Miller and Rollnick (1991) point out that it is actually a function of the patient-therapist interaction. They suggest "motivational interviewing," a technique based upon five general principles: validating ambivalence, which is a normal stage in the recovery process; increasing cognitive dissonance in the patient's perception of dual diagnosis problems, which will move the therapeutic process into a contemplation stage; avoiding argumentation and labeling, which can actually solidify resistance; "rolling" with resistance by encouraging the patient to examine problems from a different perspective; and building self-efficacy through optimism and collaborative problem solving. The clinician is also encouraged to focus on objective data rather than adopt a confrontational stance.

Support. The second principle of brief inpatient treatment of dual diagnosis patients is a supportive therapeutic stance. Dual diagnosis patients appear less able to tolerate confrontational, high-intensity treatment than those who are primarily addicted to substances (Evans and Sullivan, 1990). This is particularly true of schizophrenic patients. Such patients are often unable to adapt to the rigors of a highly structured and intensive treatment programs. Instead, the primary emphasis should be placed upon repetition, orientation to the treatment environment, education about dual diagnoses, development of interpersonal skills, cognitive restructuring, an acknowledgment that progress will be gradual, and education of the patient's family about the particular challenges of dual diagnoses (Evans and Sullivan, 1990; Group for the Advancement of Psychiatry Committee on Alcoholism and the Addictions, 1991).

Multidisciplinary intervention. This principle is important due to the complexity of daily living problems that dual diagnosis patients present. Since both addictive and psychiatric disorders have biological, psychological, and social components (Chiauzzi, 1991; Engel, 1977), it is imperative that brief inpatient treatments of these patients involve psychiatrists in conjunction with psychologists, social workers, addiction counselors, and nurses. Many of these patients present with case management problems such as inadequate housing, meager social support, lack of transportation, and poor money-handling skills. These factors can increase the likelihood of relapse with both disorders and need aggressive attention, particularly in a short-term inpatient stay.

Utilization of self-help groups. This component is even more critical for dual diagnosis patients than purely addicted patients, because of their frequent disconnection from normal avenues of social support. Attendance at Alcoholics Anonymous or Narcotics Anonymous is routinely included in treatment plans of dual diagnosis patients and has definite advantages—the support such groups provide can assist in both psychiatric and addiction treatment goals, particularly relapse prevention; the hopeful messages and testimonials of group members can build self-efficacy; the group rules and guidelines can help dual diagnosis patients develop structure in their lives; the twelve-step groups present an opportunity for social skill building; and the ready availability of these groups enables patients to rely on a diversified support system.

However, attendance at groups is not so simple for those who feel overwhelmed in a group setting or who have difficulties with self-disclosure. Reactions to self-help groups may vary by diagnosis. Depressed individuals who exhibit chronic guilt may be told that they are "sitting on the pity pot." "Drunkalogues" given by recovering A.A. speakers may inadvertently trigger unwanted memories in posttraumatic stress disorder patients. The paranoid patient may envision retribution by fellow A.A. members if he discloses personal information.

As a result, dual diagnosis patients require a flexible approach to self-help groups (Chiauzzi and Liljegren, 1993). Maximum information should be given, including the format and expectations of twelve-step meetings, since they are often confusing to newcomers; relevant literature (for example, the "Big Book") that describes the philosophy of these groups; practice in skills that enhance group involvement, for example, conversational and self-disclosure skills; the debunking of myths about self-help groups (for example, that they engage in brainwashing or seek to recruit people into cults or religions); and descriptions of different types of meetings (speaker, discussion, step, open, closed, and so on), so that the patient can develop a comfortable combination. The latter point is especially critical, as many patients assume that large speaker meetings are the only type of meeting when they can also choose from smaller, discussion-oriented meetings.

Relapse Prevention with Specific Psychiatric Disorders

Depending on the specific comorbid psychiatric disorder, certain treatment approaches may be differentially effective in preventing relapse.

Depression. The first consideration in relapse prevention relates to the potential for suicide, particularly when alcohol use is involved. The Group for the Advancement of Psychiatry Committee on Alcoholism and the Addictions (1991) cites these three significant findings: the lifetime risk of suicide among alcoholics is about 15 percent; alcohol abuse is a factor in about 25 to 50 percent of suicides; and the first and second risk factors for suicide in the general population are depression and alcohol use. Depressed substance abusers often deny suicidal tendencies while abstinent, but substance use can lower their behavioral controls over their self-destructive urges. Clinicians should therefore identify high-risk situations for substance use *and* suicidal behavior.

Relapse prevention should be a routine component of treatment for depressed addicted patients because treatment gains erode over time. About 20 percent of depressed patients relapse by six months, 40 percent by twelve months, and 50 percent by twenty-four months (Lavori, Keller, and Klerman, 1984). The major predictors of depression relapse are the number of previous episodes; the frequency of major life events; and a high level of expressed negative emotion by family members (Wilson, 1992). High-quality social support and identification of pleasant events to counter negative life events can act as buffers against relapse with these patients.

Anxiety Disorders. The course of an anxiety disorder is typified by periodic exacerbations and remissions (Barlow, 1988). The relapse rates with medications such as imipramine are approximately 35 to 40 percent, while about 25 to 40 percent of patients fail to respond to behavioral treatments such as cognitive-behavioral therapy (Brown and Barlow, 1992). Anticipatory anxiety and avoidance behavior are frequent even when the therapeutic response is positive. As a result, the treatment outcome with anxiety should be regarded differently than the treatment outcome with addiction, as complete abstinence may not be possible. The family therapy component of anxiety treatment may improve outcome, since it may prevent patient dropout and facilitate practice of anxiety-reduction (exposure to arousing situations, relaxation) skills (Brown and Barlow, 1992).

The most challenging consideration in treating the anxious addicted patient is the addictive nature of minor tranquilizers (Zweben and Smith, 1989). Not only do addiction-prone individuals have high potential for abusing benzodiazepines, but they may experience a withdrawal syndrome even with cessation of low dosages within a therapeutic range (Zweben and Smith, 1989). Nonaddictive alternatives such as the anxiolytic buspirone, tricyclic antidepressants, and psychological interventions should therefore be explored. The use of an exposure-based behavioral treatment (Barlow, 1988) or the cognitive therapy approach of Beck and Emery (1985) offers effective and less risky possibilities.

Schizophrenia. The severe psychiatric symptoms of schizophrenics often overshadow their substance abuse problems. Favorable prognostic indicators such as cognitive skills, social support, insight, stimulating activities, stable living arrangements, motivation, and employment are often lacking in schizophrenics. Social pressure, craving, and intense underlying emotions can increase a tendency to self-medicate. Due to their high relapse risk, addicted schizophrenics require treatment that is flexible, comprehensive, multidimensional, and long term (Drake, McLaughlin, Pepper, and Minkoff, 1991). For instance, schizophrenics may not readily agree to abstinence from substances and may require a longer period of engagement before they submit to addiction treatment (Mueser, Bellack, and Blanchard, 1992). Confrontation and the traditional prohibition in recovery of all mind-altering substances (including psychotropic medication) are not appropriate for this population, since such interventions may increase intense and unmanageable affect. Support, empathy, education, skill building, and social interaction should be emphasized and can be facilitated by twelve-step involvement. Earlier suggestions regarding the twelve-step component of treatment are especially applicable to addicted schizophrenics.

Personality Disorders. Personality disorders are frequently ignored in dual diagnosis treatment but can contribute significantly to relapse (Chiauzzi and Liljegren, 1993). An understanding of the relationship between personality styles and addiction can increase clinicians' predictive abilities. The style of an addicted patient's relapse and treatment response can conform to his or her personality style. Antisocial personalities may reject the expectations of A.A. peers and therapists; paranoid personalities may feel hypervigilant; dependent personalities may not take responsibility for their recoveries; passive-aggressive personalities may harbor resentments; avoidant personalities may feel self-conscious in groups of people, and compulsive personalities may ignore feelings and become excessively task oriented in recovery. It is therefore critical to evaluate Axis II as well as Axis I disorders in dual diagnosis treatment (Blume, 1989).

Conclusion

In summary, although the treatment of the dual diagnosis patient adds substantial increased complexity to inpatient care, there is a body of knowledge and clear empirically based principles, which are available to guide and direct this care.

References

Barlow, D. H. *Anxiety and Its Disorders: The Nature and Treatment of Anxiety and Panic.* New York: Guilford Press, 1988.

Beck, A. T., and Emery, G. *Anxiety Disorders and Phobias: A Cognitive Perspective.* New York: Basic Books, 1985.

Blume, S. B. "Dual Diagnosis: Psychoactive Substance Dependence and the Personality Disorders." *Journal of Psychoactive Drugs,* 1989, *21,* 139–144.

Brown, S. A., and Schuckit, M. A. "Changes in Depression Among Abstinent Alcoholics." *Journal of Studies on Alcohol,* 1988, *49,* 412–417.

Brown, T. A., and Barlow, D. H. "Panic Disorder and Panic Disorder with Agoraphobia." In P. H. Wilson (ed.), *Principles and Practice of Relapse Prevention.* New York: Guilford Press, 1992.

Bukstein, O. G., Brent, D. A., and Kaminer, Y. "Comorbidity of Substance Abuse and Other Psychiatric Disorders in Adolescents." *American Journal of Psychiatry,* 1989, *146,* 1131–1141.

Chiauzzi, E. J. *Preventing Relapse in the Addictions: A Biopsychosocial Approach.* Elmsford, N.Y.: Pergamon Press, 1991.

Chiauzzi, E. J., and Liljegren, S. E. "Taboo Topics in Addictions Treatment: An Empirical Review of Clinical Folklore." *Journal of Substance Abuse Treatment,* 1993, *10,* 303–316.

Cox, B. J., Norton, G. R., Swinson, R. P., and Endler, N. S. "Substance Abuse and Panic-Related Anxiety: A Critical Review." *Behavior Research and Therapy,* 1990, *28,* 385–393.

De Soto, C. B., O'Donnell, W. E., Allred, L. J., and Lopes, C. E. "Symptomatology in Alcoholics at Various Stages of Abstinence." *Alcoholism: Clinical and Experimental Research,* 1985, *9,* 505–512.

DiClemente, C. C. "Motivational Interviewing and the Stages of Change." In W. R. Miller and S. Rollnick (eds.), *Motivational Interviewing: Preparing People to Change Addictive Behavior.* New York: Guilford Press, 1991.

Drake, R. E., McLaughlin, P., Pepper, B., and Minkoff, K. "Dual Diagnosis of Major Mental Illness and Substance Disorder: An Overview." In K. Minkoff and R. Drake (eds.), *Dual Diagnosis of Major Mental Illness and Substance Disorder.* New Directions for Mental Health Services, no. 50. San Francisco: Jossey-Bass, 1991.

Engel, G. L. "The Need for a New Medical Model: A Challenge for Biomedicine." *Science,* 1977, *196,* 129–136.

Evans, K., and Sullivan, J. M. *Dual Diagnosis: Counseling the Mentally Ill Substance Abuser.* New York: Guilford Press, 1990.

Group for the Advancement of Psychiatry Committee on Alcoholism and the Addictions. "Substance Abuse Disorders: A Psychiatric Priority." *American Journal of Psychiatry,* 1991, *148,* 1291–1300.

Helzer, J. E., and Pryzbeck, T. R. "The Co-occurrence of Alcoholism with Other Psychiatric Disorders in the General Population and Its Impact on Treatment." *Journal of Studies on Alcohol,* 1988, *49,* 219–224.

Kosten, T. R., and Kleber, H. D. "Differential Diagnosis of Psychiatric Comorbidity in Substance Abusers." *Journal of Substance Abuse Treatment,* 1988, *5,* 201–206.

Lavori, P. W., Keller, M. B., and Klerman, G. L. "Relapse in Affective Disorders: A Reanalysis of the Literature Using Life Table Methods." *Journal of Psychiatric Research,* 1984, *18,* 13–25.

McCrady, B. S., and Smith, D. E. "Implications of Cognitive Impairment for the Treatment of Alcoholism." *Alcoholism: Clinical and Experimental Research,* 1986, *10,* 145–149.

McLellan, A. T., Luborsky, L., Woody, G. E., O'Brien, C. P., and Druley, K. A. "Predicting Response to Alcohol and Drug Abuse Treatments." *Archives of General Psychiatry,* 1983, *40,* 620–625.

Meyer, R. E. (ed.). *Psychopathology and Addictive Disorders.* New York: Guilford Press, 1986.

Miller, W. R. "Motivation for Treatment: A Review with Special Emphasis on Alcoholism." *Psychological Bulletin,* 1985, *98,* 84–107.

Miller, W. R., and Rollnick, S. (eds). *Motivational Interviewing: Preparing People to Change Addictive Behavior.* New York: Guilford Press, 1991.

Minkoff, K. "Program Components of a Comprehensive Integrated Care System for Serious Mentally Ill Patients with Substance Disorders." In K. Minkoff and R. Drake (eds.), *Dual Diagnosis of Major Mental Illness and Substance Disorder.* New Directions for Mental Health Services, no. 50. San Francisco: Jossey-Bass, 1991.

Mirin, S. M., and Weiss, R. D. "Substance Abuse and Mental Illness." In R. J. Frances and S. I. Miller (eds.), *Clinical Textbook of Addictive Disorders.* New York: Guilford Press, 1991.

Mueser, K. T., Bellack, A. S., and Blanchard, J. J. "Comorbidity of Schizophrenia and Substance Abuse: Implications for Treatment." *Journal of Consulting and Clinical Psychology,* 1992, *60,* 845–856.

Nace, E. P., Davis, C. W., and Gaspari, J. P. "Axis II Comorbidity in Substance Abusers." *American Journal of Psychiatry,* 1991, *148,* 118–120.

Ross, H. E., Glaser, F. B., and Germanson, T. "The Prevalence of Psychiatric Disorders in Patients with Alcohol and Other Drug Problems." *Archives of General Psychiatry,* 1988, *45,* 1023–1031.

Rounsaville, B. J., Weissman, M. M., Kleber, H., and Wilber, C. "Heterogeneity of Psychiatric Diagnosis in Treated Opiate Addicts." *Archives of General Psychiatry,* 1982, *33,* 161–166.

Schneier, F. R., and Siris, S. G. "A Review of Psychoactive Substance Use and Abuse in Schizophrenia: Patterns of Drug Choice. *Journal of Nervous and Mental Disease,* 1987, *175,* 641–652.

Tarter, R. E., Ott, P. J., and Mezzich, A. C. "Psychometric Assessment." In R. J. Frances and S. I. Miller (eds.), *Clinical Textbook of Addictive Disorders.* New York: Guilford Press, 1991.

Vaillant, G. E. "Is Alcoholism More Often the Cause or the Result of Depression?" *Harvard Review of Psychiatry,* July/Aug. 1993, pp. 94–99.

Weiss, K. J., and Rosenberg, D. J. "Prevalence of Anxiety Disorder Among Alcoholics." *Journal of Clinical Psychiatry,* 1985, *46,* 3–5.

Wilson, P. H. "Depression." In P. H. Wilson (ed.), *Principles and Practice of Relapse Prevention.* New York: Guilford Press, 1992.

Zweben, J. E., and Smith, D. E. "Considerations in Using Psychotropic Medications with Dual Diagnosis Patients in Recovery." *Journal of Psychoactive Drugs,* 1989, *21,* 221–228.

EMIL CHIAUZZI, Ph.D., is clinical director of the Addictions Treatment Program at Waltham Weston Hospital, in Waltham, Massachusetts.

Some common medical conditions, recommended treatment regimens, and situations in which a patient may require transfer to an acute medical facility are described for the inpatient psychiatrist facing ever more patients who have comorbid medical and psychiatric disabilities.

Medical Problems in Hospitalized Psychiatric Patients

Susan J. Fiester, Michael M. Shefferman

The evaluation and/or treatment of a medical problem is often a critical aspect of a patient's overall care while he or she is receiving psychiatric hospitalization. Although another physician (for example, the internist, family practitioner, or gynecologist) may be available for consultation and advice, the attending psychiatrist is ultimately responsible for the care of the patient, including the patient's medical problems. Although the psychiatrist is not likely to have, and in fact, does not need to have, certain specific types of medical expertise, it is important that he or she have a grasp of some general guiding principles for the medical care of the hospitalized psychiatric patient.

Medical care of a hospitalized patient begins with the admission medical history and physical examination. This is preferably performed by an internist but in some cases may be done by the attending psychiatrist. Although the medical history and physical examination are sometimes looked upon as ancillary to the true focus on the patient's psychiatric care, they are a vital aspect of the patient's hospitalization. They function as a complete screening assessment of the patient's physical status and should include funduscopic examination, neurological examination, and where appropriate, genital and rectal examinations. The medical history and physical examination together with the initial psychiatric, nursing, and psychosocial assessments form the cornerstone for developing the initial treatment plan for the patient.

Attention to the patient's physical status has four principal aims:

To identify and treat underlying medical problems that might be etiologically related to some or all of the psychiatric problems. Some examples of the many disorders that can cause significant psychiatric symptoms include hypothyroidism, CNS tumor, hypercalcemia, and acute intermittent porphyria.

To identify and treat medical problems that, although not etiologically related to the psychiatric problem, may be making significant contributions to the patient's psychiatric condition. Examples include most chronic disabling diseases, such as heart disease or diabetes.

To identify and treat illnesses with physical or physiological components that require accurate diagnosis and management of both the psychological and physical symptoms, such as the anxiety disorders or somatization disorders.

To identify existing medical problems that require parallel management during the patient's psychiatric hospitalization and treatment but are not contributing significantly or negatively to the patient's psychiatric clinical status or current acute psychiatric problem. Examples include hypertension and cardiac arrhythmia.

To protect the public health of the hospital community by identification and control of contagious diseases.

Since free-standing psychiatric hospitals and psychiatric units in many general hospitals are not equipped to provide specialized medical care, decisions must often be made regarding the medical appropriateness of a patient's admission and treatment in a psychiatric unit. In general, if a patient's medical problems prohibit participation in the psychiatric treatment regimen, treatment on a psychiatric unit is inappropriate. For the most part, the medical problems treated in the context of a psychiatric hospitalization are likely to be more similar to those treated in an outpatient practitioner's office than to those treated in a medical-surgical hospital.

If, subsequent to admission, a new medical problem is diagnosed, the attending psychiatrist, in consultation with the hospital internist, must decide whether the problem can be adequately managed or whether a specialist should be consulted. Frequently, specialty consultation can be deferred until after the patient is discharged. If the patient has not been under the care of a primary physician, the attending psychiatrist should provide the patient with resources for referral and follow-up care.

In addition to identifying and treating medical problems in the psychiatric patient, the in-hospital setting presents an opportunity to educate the patient about his or her medical illness and its management, through discussions with nursing or medical staff and provision of educational materials. The physician may also choose to review with the patient risk factors for disease (such as cigarette smoking), life-style factors that influence disease (such as activity level and diet), and preventive medical care. Specific interventions may also be provided such as smoking-cessation programs, dietary consultations for weight reduction or management, and activities therapy consultations for developing appropriate exercise regimens.

Common Medical Problems

Medical care of psychiatric inpatients does require some basic knowledge and understanding of medical problems, but what it requires most is a commonsense approach. We will make no attempt here to condense a textbook of medicine into one chapter but rather will attempt to present a basic knowledge foundation with which psychiatrists should be familiar and to outline a commonsense approach to the management of the most frequent and troublesome medical problems that will be encountered in psychiatric inpatients.

Diabetes Mellitus. (This section is based on Rifkin, 1989, and O'Hare and Weir, 1990.) When selecting a treatment for a medical problem, medical students are often taught to elicit a history of what treatments the patient has previously received and how he or she has responded: "If it worked, do it again. If it didn't, don't." Nowhere is this approach more appropriate than in the management of diabetic patients in a psychiatric hospital. An enormous body of medical literature presents novel and highly effective regimens for optimal blood glucose control in diabetic patients over the long term. However, in an era of brief hospital stays and focused treatment, psychiatrists must not lose sight of the necessary focus on the short-term rather than long-term management of the patient's medical problems. The aim is to provide stabilization for acute problems and/or adequately manage medical problems until the patient can return to the long-term care of his or her physician.

If the patient's blood glucose level is reasonably well controlled, continue with the current diabetic regimen (diet, oral agent, insulin, and so forth) even if the particular regimen does not necessary reflect the optimal approach or the approach the hospital internist or psychiatrist would use in long-term management. Diabetic patients who are comfortable with their usual form of management may have a difficult time radically altering their regimens, and attempts at radical alterations of the regimen may result in unstable (high or low) glucose levels, which might ultimately distract attention from the primary focus on treating the patient's psychiatric problems.

If a diabetic patient is poorly controlled, the best approach is to stop all long-acting insulin and prescribe scheduled doses of regular insulin based on finger stick glucose levels four times daily, for example, at 7:00 A.M., 11:30 A.M., 4:30 P.M., and 10:00 P.M. This same approach can be used for a newly diagnosed diabetic or a diabetic on oral hypoglycemics whose blood glucose levels can not be adequately controlled without insulin. With this approach, in addition to gaining control of the patient's blood glucose level on an immediate basis, the physician can also determine how much total regular insulin the patient is requiring in one day, in order to estimate the amount of long-acting insulin required. The patient can then be shifted to a long-acting insulin regimen.

In considering the meaning of blood glucose control in the context of short-term caretaking, it is important to note that hypoglycemia can kill in a matter of minutes but hyperglycemia can be tolerated for much longer periods without significant problems. Low blood glucose levels can be extremely dangerous as some acutely ill psychiatric patients may not be able to recognize the subtle symptoms that precede a serious hypoglycemic episode. It may be preferable to maintain blood sugars slightly higher than one might otherwise. Therefore, "control," in the case of the psychiatric inpatient, might mean blood sugars no higher than 200 mg percent, but not in the range that would be considered normal for the general diabetic population.

Identification of serious *acute* lack of control of diabetes does not depend solely on blood sugar levels; however, persistent blood sugar levels above 300 mg percent are of concern. Evidence of significant ketosis (3+ to 4+) in the urine and clinical signs and symptoms of impending ketoacidotic coma (obtundation, tachycardia, tachypnea, odor of acetone on the breath) are reasons for immediate transfer to a medical facility for emergency treatment.

Obtaining a glycosololated hemoglobin level may also provide an indication of how well controlled the patient's blood glucose has been over the past several months. This information can be presented to the patient as positive reinforcement for good compliance with his or her current diabetic regimen or as feedback about problems with compliance and encouragement for improvement in the future.

Hypertension. (This section is based on Fletcher and Bulpitt, 1992, and Maheswarau, Gill, Davieo, and others, 1991.) Measuring blood pressure in the usual clinical setting with a sphygmomanometer provides only an indirect estimate of blood pressure. The only direct measure of mean arterial blood pressure is a reading from an arterial catheter. Too much emphasis is often placed on a single reading taken in the hospital setting with the possibility of inaccuracies in measurement. In addition, blood pressure is subject to momentary dramatic fluctuations. Substantial short-term elevation can be caused by emotional states such as anger, fear, anxiety, and frustration, which may be particularly likely to be experienced by hospitalized psychiatric patients.

Hypertensive cardiovascular disease is characterized by sustained elevated blood pressure (especially diastolic) which can lead to serious vascular sequelae over time. Hypertensive cardiovascular disease rarely presents at a level of severity that requires acute emergency intervention (accelerated or malignant hypertension). Although hospitalized psychiatric patients frequently have elevated blood pressure, sometimes alarmingly so, they seldom have elevated blood pressure that requires immediate acute treatment with antihypertensive medication.

As with diabetes mellitus, it is important to distinguish between the short-term management of the problem and the long-term definitive treatment. The goal of antihypertensive treatment is the reduction of long-term risks rather than the treatment of single blood pressure recordings. Clearly, the immediate risk of overcontrol or excessive reduction of blood pressure is the creation of hypotension. This potential is even greater in the psychiatric population, where patients are frequently being treated with psychotropic medications that cause significant orthostatic changes.

Accelerated or malignant hypertension, the only true hypertensive emergency, is characterized by severe retinal changes including papilledema, evidence of encephalopathy, renal dysfunction, EKG abnormalities, and even congestive heart failure. Consistently elevated blood pressure readings in the range of 200/120 or above should trigger further investigation to determine if the physical findings or laboratory results noted above are present. Elevated blood pressure alone does not constitute malignant hypertension. If malignant hypertension exists, the patient should be transferred to an acute medical facility for immediate treatment.

Treatment of patients with elevated blood pressure but not malignant hypertension involves repeated monitoring of the blood pressure at least two or three times daily for three or four days or more, depending on the blood pressure level. Based on the series of blood pressure readings, decisions can be made about whether the patient requires antihypertensive medication or can be managed with a program of life-style alterations including weight loss, restricted sodium diet, exercise and stress management, and relaxation techniques. This process is especially important for patients going through active detoxification from alcohol or other substances. No determination should be made about the presence or absence of long-term hypertension until the detoxification has been completed. More often than not, blood pressure, although sometimes dramatically elevated during detoxification, returns to normal after patients finish detoxification or as their psychiatric status stabilizes. Patients in an acute psychiatric state (for example, acute psychosis, acute mania, or acute anxiety) should also be stabilized before making a decision to institute medical treatment for hypertension. If there are still significant elevations of blood pressure on a consistent basis when the patient is stable (for example, diastolic blood pressure of greater than 100 mm Hq or systolic blood pressure greater than 150 mm Hq), antihypertensive medication should be instituted. Either an angiotensin converting enzyme (ACE) inhibitor or a thiazide diuretic could be the initial agent of choice. If the patient's blood pressure is between 90 to 100 diastolic or 130 to 150 systolic, antihypertensive therapy does not need to be instituted, but the patient should be referred for follow-up with an internist after discharge.

Headaches. (This section is based on Headache Classification Committee, 1988, and Linet and others, 1989.) Headaches are among the most common complaints in nearly every specialty area of medicine. Although it is clearly important to identify those cases of headache caused by organic disorders (brain tumors, encephalopathy, hematomata) that may occur in a psychiatrically ill patient, the overwhelming number of headaches are not caused by serious organic disorders but can be classified into two primary categories: vasoreactive (migraine) and muscle/tension headaches. These are more often the effect of the underlying psychiatric disorder than a cause thereof, as a brain tumor might be. In cases of migraine or tension headache, the history and physical examination findings are typical of the disorders. There is an absence of significant neurological findings and special studies such as CAT scans or magnetic resonance imaging (MRI) are not indicated.

In the treatment of the benign headaches, it is very important to avoid creating the iatrogenic problems of analgesic abuse or dependence. This can often be a difficult path as one of the commonly used treatments for migraine contains butalbital and as narcotic analgesics are often requested by the patient and prescribed. It is also important to avoid problematic interaction of medications used to treat headaches with other medications, especially psychotropic medications. The nonsteroidal antiinflammatory drugs (NSAIDs), not without potential problems of their own, have proven very useful in treating migraine and tension headaches. The recent availability of sumatriptan for treating acute migraine episodes is a significant advance as is the availability of Toradol, a new injectable and potent NSAID. In general, if the headaches have been a chronic problem that the patient has managed with a particular regimen, continuing that regimen may be most appropriate even if the psychiatrist feels that it might not represent the ultimate management regimen for severe chronic headache. Referral after discharge to a specialty outpatient chronic pain treatment program may be indicated.

Most of all, the headaches ought not be permitted to become the major focus of the patient's treatment, allowing him or her to avoid attention to the underlying psychiatric problems.

Chest Pain. (This section is based on Carney, Freedland, Rich, and Jaffe, 1991; Chiquan, Lepine, and Ades, 1993; and Yingling, Wulsin, Arnold, and Rovan, 1993). The practice of medicine is learned in academic medical centers and their affiliated teaching hospitals. Most physicians learn about chest pain by caring for patients who have coronary artery disease or other serious heart or lung disease. But outside the coronary care unit, coronary artery disease is the far less common cause of chest pain. Psychiatrists are also likely to see patients with complaints of chest pain, as chest pain is a commonly occurring symptom of panic disorder and other anxiety states. In addition, chest pain related to chest wall muscle strain and/or costochondral junction and intercostal muscle injury is as common in psychiatrically ill patients as it is in the general population. Few of the episodes of chest pain one is likely to encounter in hospitalized psychiatric patients will require a stat EKG or transfer to an emergency room for evaluation.

Upper G.I. Disease. (This discussion is based on Drossman, 1991.) Because of the effects of substances of abuse, especially alcohol, and of many medications on the pathophysiology and function of the upper gastrointestinal tract, psychiatrists caring for hospitalized patients are likely to confront symptoms of peptic ulcer disease, gastroesophageal reflux disease, and symptomatic hiatal hernia. Epigastric and retrosternal burning discomfort are generally easy to recognize, but the pain of esophageal spasm which may accompany them may be very difficult to distinguish from the pain of coronary artery disease.

If the problem has been previously evaluated and identified, the best course of action, once again, is to continue whatever regimen has been successful in the past. Additionally, in previously diagnosed patients with active symptoms, especially alcohol abusers, at least three stools should be screened for the presence of occult blood to ensure there is no active bleeding from the upper G.I. tract.

If the problem has not been previously diagnosed and there is no evidence of active bleeding or perforation, it is reasonable to treat the patient symptomatically with antacids or acid secretion inhibitors (histamine 2 receptor antagonists) and arrange for a G.I. evaluation (for example, upper endoscopy or upper G.I. radiography), if indicated, after the patient is discharged.

Irritable Bowel (Spastic Colon) Syndrome. (This discussion is based on Guthrie, Creed, Dawson, and Tomenson, 1991, and Walker, Roy-Byrne, and Katon, 1990). Although its etiology and pathophysiology now appear to be more complex than once believed, irritable bowel syndrome can still be thought of as a hyperreactive state in which there is exaggeration of the normal physiological process. The signs and symptoms are what might be expected from hyperperistalsis: increased gas, bloating, gurgling, nausea, uncomfortable spasms, abdominal pain, diarrhea and/or constipation (sometimes alternating), plus palpably tight (spastic) and tender colon at any or all points of its course around the abdomen. Several specific causes have been identified including some foods and medications and intestinal lactose sensitivity, but it is such a commonplace reaction to "stress" that there should be no surprise at encountering it frequently it in a psychiatric hospital.

Dehydration (even very mild) and lack of fiber in the diet are precipitants or aggravators of the problem and can be corrected by attention to the patient's oral fluid intake and by addition of high fiber foods to his or her diet and/or supplements of fiber. Mild anticholinergic agents such as the belladonna alkaloids and mild antianxiety agents can be useful, but care must be taken not to add to the anticholinergic and sedative side effects of many psychotropic agents. In fact, sometimes those very side effects are helpful in "treating" the G.I. symptoms.

Though it can be extremely uncomfortable and distressing, no one has yet died of spastic colon syndrome. Therefore, our mainstays of treatment are oral fluids, increased dietary or supplementary fiber, and patient education and reassurance.

Thyroid Dysfunction. (This discussion is based on Bakerman, 1984, and Helfand and Cvapo, 1990). The clinical recognition of thyroid dysfunction is complicated by the great overlap of signs and symptoms between hyperthyroidism and anxiety and between hypothyroidism and depression. Yet the majority of diagnostic errors in psychiatric patients are made because of misinterpretation of laboratory tests. There is no single thyroid test that, by itself, can reliably indicate thyroid function. The two most commonly used screening tests (T3 uptake and T4 by RIA) are useful because they are complementary, but they are subject to factitious alterations resulting from the presence of estrogens (oral contraceptives, pregnancy, postmenopausal estrogen replacement, or liver disease), protein binding medications (such as carbamazepine), and concurrent disease.

The most useful tests for screening of thyroid function are the T3 uptake, T4, and T7 (or Free Thyroxine Index, which is calculated from the T3 and T4 results). An abnormally low value for any of these screening tests should be followed by a thyroid stimulating hormone (TSH) level. Confirmed TSH levels above 20 microunits/ml leave little question of the existence of primary hypothyroidism. However, levels above the upper limits of normal (usually in the 5.5 area) but less than 20 are more difficult to interpret. Many consider these levels to represent occult hypothyroidism and recommend treatment with thyroid supplements.

Since the thyroid gland and hypothalamus operate in a direct feedback mechanism, a patient cannot be injured by receiving thyroid supplements even if he or she does not really need them as long as the dose is no more than the average full suppressive dose.

Liver Disease (and What Isn't Liver Disease). (This discussion is based on Boyer and Miller, 1987, and Berg and Tryding, 1981). The presence of positive antibodies to hepatitis B and hepatitis C is extremely commonplace in intravenous drug abusers. This serves as evidence that the patient has been infected with a hepatitis virus and has become "immune" through the development of antibodies. Many other patients have evidence of chronic hepatitis without specific antibodies (non-A, non-B hepatitis). All, however, usually reflect a benign low-grade chronic form of disease, which more often causes discomfort for the treating physician and treatment team than for the patient. During the acute infection period, following the universal precautions is a must. It is unusual for hepatitis B to present other clinical concerns on a psychiatric unit, and the degree of liver dysfunction is rarely enough to pose an absolute contraindication to the use of most psychotropic drugs. A patient with severely compromised liver disease function (hepatic failure) resulting from any etiology should not be treated on a psychiatric unit.

The same observations are true for patients with alcoholic liver disease. In most instances, the acute changes in liver function of alcoholic liver disease (elevated liver enzyme tests) will resolve uneventfully as the patient remains abstinent from alcohol. However, acute hepatic encephalopathy is another medical emergency that requires transfer of the patient to an acute medical facility. The diagnosis is made by the clinical appearance of the patient, not by serum ammonia levels. Likewise, acute delirium tremens (not just "the shakes") is a clinically diagnosed medical emergency that requires intravenous fluids and an acute medical care facility.

Since it is common to perform screening tests of liver function in psychiatric inpatient units, two frequent situations arise where isolated test abnormalities may be inadvertently viewed as evidence of liver disease. This misperception can lead to delays in initiating needed psychotropic agents. The first of these situations is Gilbert's syndrome, which is a congenital deficiency of the enzyme that facilitates the conversion of insoluble to soluble bilirubin, leading to an increase in the level of total bilirubin in the blood. All other liver function tests are normal, and the patient's liver function in all other respects is normal. The bilirubin level may be quite variable, ranging from normal to an elevation substantial enough to cause mild clinical jaundice and a mistaken diagnosis of hepatitis. Gilbert's syndrome is quite common and benign and does not require specific treatment.

Gamma glutamyl transpeptidase (GGTP) is an enzyme made by the liver that is often measured along with others as part of the liver function tests. Its principal value is in distinguishing elevations of alkaline phosphatase caused by liver problems that are caused by bone disease. Alkaline phosphatase is present in both liver and bone, but GGTP is present only in the liver and arises from the same site on the liver cell as does alkaline phosphatase. That site on the hepatocellular membrane is also the site of binding of alcohol, cocaine, opioids, and many medications, including all of the anticonvulsants such as phenytoin, carbamazepine, valproic acid, and the barbiturates. All of those substances (and others) have a high incidence of causing false positive elevations of GGTP. Elevated GGTP resulting from alcohol intake persists for some time after ingestion and has been used by some to monitor alcohol relapse. Elevated GGTP in the face of otherwise normal liver function tests is nearly always due to one or more of the above circumstances and should not be looked upon as evidence of liver disease.

Syphilis and Tuberculosis: "It Can't Happen Here." (This discussion is based on Romanski and others, 1991, and Centers for Disease Control, 1990.) Though the media currently suggest otherwise, tuberculosis and syphilis have not returned—they never left. And, as with all other infections, the emergence of HIV disease has magnified the problem. Some jurisdictions are compelled by law to screen all admissions to the hospital for syphilis, in order to detect otherwise undiagnosed cases of active disease. However, it can sometimes be difficult to correctly interpret the positive syphilis serologies that are related to previously treated disease or the biological false positives that are frequent in intravenous drug users. Once the diagnosis of syphilis is properly made, treatment should be carried out according to Centers for Disease Control recommendations. Additionally, the local health department must be notified.

Tuberculosis has become more of a problem because of the emergence of many treatment-resistant strains. The mission of the psychiatric hospital should be to rapidly screen staff as well as new patients for evidence of active tuberculosis. Skin testing (PPD) is a valuable prospective screening tool for large populations, but it requires physicians to obtain a definitive reading and has too much built-in delay for rapid screening of new patients for active disease. Therefore, at least a single view chest X ray should be performed on every adult nonpregnant inpatient who has not had one in the previous ten months. Any others, including children, whose history or examination suggests the possibility of active tuberculosis should also receive a chest X ray. A patient with a positive PPD and a negative chest X ray should have an internal medicine consultation, to consider the positives and negatives of prophylactic antituberculous medication. The health department must also be notified and consideration should be given to family members and residents of the household having screening PPDs.

A patient with newly diagnosed active tuberculosis should be immediately isolated and placed on respiratory precautions and transferred to a medical facility as soon as possible for further evaluation and initiation of treatment. Current necessities for physically isolating an infected patient and his or her room are beyond the mission of a psychiatric hospital. The patient ought not return to the psychiatric facility until his or her sputa are negative for tuberculosis organisms.

HIV Disease. Complete discussion of HIV disease would require more pages than this entire chapter. The unfortunate increase in the prevalence of the disease generally will be reflected in psychiatric hospital populations as well and using the universal precautions is critical for the protection of all. HIV encephalopathy and psychosis will make psychiatric hospitals necessary foci of the evaluation and treatment of such patients. In addition, the depression and substance abuse that are frequently concurrent with HIV disease will necessarily keep psychiatric hospitals in the battle.

As long as a patient is not actively shedding virus through open bleeding, severe diarrhea, open sores, and so forth, there is no reason why he or she cannot be managed on a psychiatric unit. If the patient is not already under the follow-up care of a physician experienced in the care of HIV disease, a consultation should be sought. The question of universal screening for the HIV antibody remains controversial but the proper use of universal precautions obviates the need for that in regard to protecting the public health of the facility. Matters of confidentiality and need for consent to testing vary among jurisdictions.

Laboratory Testing

In the "old days," psychiatrists had very little interest in laboratory testing, but with the recognition of the biological and chemical nature of psychiatric illness, the pendulum has swung the other way in many respects. Thus, it is important to distinguish the importance of and usefulness of screening tests as opposed to more definitive testing. Screening tests are those that are relatively quick and easy to do for the laboratory, have a reasonable likelihood of identifying for the physician some fairly common condition that might otherwise be missed, and are relatively inexpensive for the patient. Each of us may see one case of Wilson's disease in our life times, but that is certainly not a good reason to screen every patient for serum copper and ceruloplasmin levels. Likewise, encephalopathy due to vitamin B12 deficiency may occur rarely in a psychiatric patient with no other suggestive findings, but that's not a good reason to screen every patient for vitamin B12 levels.

Electrocardiograms, MRIs, karyotyping, various blood and urine tests, and so on, can all be of great value to the psychiatrist in the management of the hospitalized patient, but their excessive and inappropriate use simply adds expense for the patient and more confusion than assistance for the physician.

Conclusion

The care and management of medical problems in the hospitalized psychiatric patient need not be an unpleasant and uncomfortable part of the territory for the psychiatrist, but it requires thoughtful use of the fund of knowledge acquired in medical school and a large dose of common sense.

References

Bakerman, S. *ABC's of Interpretive Laboratory Data* (2nd ed.). Greenville, N.C.: Interpretive Laboratory Data, 1984.

Berg, B., and Tryding, N. "False Positive Serum GGT Tests." *Lancet,* May 23, 1981, p. 1162.

Boyer, J. L., and Miller, D. J. "Chronic Hepatitis." In L. Shiff and E. R. Shiff (eds.), *Diseases of the Liver* (6th ed.). Philadelphia, PA: Lippincott, 1987.

Carney, R. M., Freedland, K. E., Rich, M. W., and Jaffe, A. S. "Psychiatric Disorders in Patients with Normal Coronary Arteries and Chest Pain." *Practical Cardiology,* 1991, *17,* 31–39.

Centers for Disease Control. "Guidelines for Preventing the Transmission of Tuberculosis in Health-Care Settings, with Special Focus on HIV-Related Issues." *Morbidity and Mortality Weekly Report,* 1990, *39,* 1–29.

Chiquan, J. M., Lepine, J. P., and Ades, J. "Panic Disorder in Cardiac Outpatients." *American Journal of Psychiatry,* 1993, *150,* 7505.

Drossman, D. A. "Psychosocial Factors in the Case of Patients with Gastrointestinal Diseases." In T. Yamada (ed.), *Textbook of Gastroenterology,* Philadelphia: Lippincott, 1991.

Fletcher, A. E., and Bulpitt, C. J. "How Far Should Blood Pressure Be Lowered?" *New England Journal of Medicine,* 1992, *326,* 251–254.

Guthrie, E., Creed, F., Dawson, D., and Tomenson, B. "A Controlled Trial of Psychological Treatment for the Irritable Bowel Syndrome. *Gastroenterology,* 1991, *100,* 450–457.

Headache Classification Committee of the International Headache Society. "Classification and Diagnostic Criteria for Headache Disorders, Cranial Neurologies and Facial Pain." *Caphalgia,* 1988, *8* (suppl. 7), 9–96.

Helfand, M., and Cvapo, L. M. "Monitoring Therapy in Patients Taking Levothyroxine." *Annals of Internal Medicine,* 1990, *113,* 450–454.

Linet, M. S., Stewart, W. F., Celetano, D. D., Ziegler, D., and Sprecher, M. "An Epidemiologic Study of Headache Among Adolescents and Young Adults." *Journal of the American Medical Association,* 1989, *261,* 2211–2216.

Maheswarau, R., Gill, J. S., Davieo, P., and others. "High Blood Pressure Due to Alcohol: A Rapidly Reversible Effect." *Hypertension,* 1991, *17,* 787–792.

O'Hare, J. A., and Weir, G. C. "Insulin Therapy." In K. L. Decker (ed.). *Principles and Practice of Endocrinology and Metabolism.* Philadelphia: Lippincott, 1990.

Rifkin, H. (ed.). *Physicians Guide to Non-Insulin Dependent (Type II) Diabetes: Diagnosis and Treatment* (2nd ed.). Alexandria, Va.: American Diabetes Association, 1989.

Romanski, B., Sutherland, R., Fick, G. M., Mooney, D., and Love, E. J. "Serologic Response to Treatment of Infectious Syphilis." *Annals of Internal Medicine*, 1991, *114*, 1005–1009.

Walker, E. A., Roy-Byrne, P. P., and Katon, W. J. "Irritable Bowel Syndrome and Psychiatric Illness." *American Journal of Psychiatry*, 1990, *147*, 565–572.

Yingling, K. W., Wulsin, L. R., Arnold, L. M., and Rovan, G. W. "Estimated Prevalences of Panic Disorder and Depression Among Consecutive Patients Seen in an Emergency Department with Acute Chest Pain." *Journal of General Internal Medicine*, 1993, *8*, 231–235.

SUSAN J. FIESTER, M.D., is medical director of the Psychiatric Institute of Washington, D.C.

MICHAEL M. SHEFFERMAN, M.D., F.A.C.P., is director of Internal Medical Services of the Psychiatric Institute of Washington, D.C., and associate clinical professor of medicine at the George Washington University School of Medicine and Health Sciences.

Most clinicians will agree that the management of the disruptive patient (and other difficult populations) poses frequent and common complications. This chapter presents key strategies and philosophies that aid the clinician in effectively treating these populations.

Managing Difficult Populations

Les Alhadeff

The very nature of psychiatric work entails having to manage difficult populations. This is especially true on the inpatient unit, where the clinician and treatment team are the patient's primary points of interaction. While this work is generally very rewarding, few would disagree it can bring with it a substantial level of strain. The particular situations and/or cases that cause a clinician difficulty undeniably vary depending on the experience, interests, and personality of the clinician. However, there are certain patient populations that are historically more difficult to manage. For instance, the treatment-resistant patient can disturb the clinician's professional self-esteem and faith in his or her abilities; similarly, the needs of the medically ill psychiatric patient or the patient with a comorbid substance abuse disorder (as discussed in Chapters Four and Five) can place a disproportionate burden on the treatment team and result in excess frustration or other difficulties.

Of particular interest, however, is the disruptive patient who exhibits impulse problems, self-destructive behaviors, pathological use of projection, or histrionic attention-seeking behaviors. Because of the frequency with which patients with a severe Axis I disorder exhibit characteristics, if not the full-blown diagnosis, of a personality disorder, this is a problem frequently encountered in the inpatient setting. Perhaps the most universally recognized difficult-to-treat patient is the borderline personality disorder (BPD). Research has suggested that as many of 63 percent of inpatients carry a comorbid borderline personality disorder, and an even greater proportion exhibit some of the characteristic borderline symptomatology (Widiger and Frances, 1989).

Because of the prevalence of this disorder in inpatient populations, and its utility in illustrating many of the difficulties encountered when working with disruptive patients, this disorder will serve as the framework for this chapter. However, in general, the information presented is broadly applicable to other populations exhibiting similar disruptive behaviors.

Disruptive Behaviors

Patients that disrupt the normal operation of a psychiatric unit do so by a myriad of strategies. Four of the more disruptive behaviors are projection, self-destruction, impulsivity, and histrionic attention-seeking behaviors.

Projection. Pathologic projection, projective identification, and poor interpersonal boundaries can create a series of disruptions, and sometimes chaos, among staff and patients on a unit. Essentially, these behaviors serve to disrupt relationships and lead to what is commonly referred to as splitting. It is often suggested that patients with these behaviors are attempting to recreate their family environments on the unit. The strong emotions evoked in the staff can lead to great difficulty in achieving a stable unified view of the patient. The intense anxiety these emotions carry leads to disruption of logical and orderly social and cognitive processes and regressed efforts at understanding. Roth (1987) observes that "counter transference in the hospital milieu is a whole topic unto itself. . . . Each of the ward recipients (various nurses, attendants, and so on) of these emotions will think he or she is the sole comprehender of the patient's 'true' emotional state. Stubborn, bitter struggles between therapist and various staff members may result" (p. 63). In borderline patients, projection can combine with a "black/white" cognitive set, resulting in even more extensive splitting among and between staff and patients. By characterizing some staff members as "good" and "kind" and others as "bad" and "unkind," and allying themselves with the "good" staff, borderline patients can create a significant chasm between these two groups. Any preexisting tension between staff members is likely to be noticed and exploited by the borderline patient. A particularly good explanation of this process is presented by Gabbard (1990):

> Staff members find themselves assuming and defending highly polarized positions against one another with a vehemence out of proportion to the importance of the issue. The patient has presented one self-representation to one group of treaters and another self-representation to another group of treaters. . . . Via projective identification, each self-representation evokes a corresponding reaction in the treater that can be understood as an unconscious identification with the projected internal object of the patient. . . . Full-blown splitting of this variety boldly illustrates the time-honored notion that patients recapitulate their internal object world in the hospital milieu. . . . Various treaters become unconsciously identified with the patient's internal objects and play out roles in a script that is written by the patient's unconscious.

Self-destruction. Suicidal and self-destructive gestures often occur at times when the patient experiences the therapist as frustrating or "not-present."

These actions, therefore, may be a manifestation of the patient's anger at this situation and his or her attempt to punish the therapist or rid the self of "badness" or other intrapsychic experiences (Gunderson, 1984). Regardless of the precise reason behind these acts, the therapist often experiences them as threatening, manipulative, and inciting rich countertransference feelings. This countertransference, coupled with the threat to the success of the treatment and the patient's life, can potentially exhaust the therapist or lead to ineffective and destructive mechanisms for dealing with the patients. For these reasons, it is often important for the therapist to set limits and a tentative stance prior to the occurrence of self-destructive acts. "The chronically suicidal borderline patient," says Gabbard (1990), "may engender intense counter transference feelings in staff members, who perceive the attempts as gestures and manipulative and therefore begin to react to the patient's suicidal threats with lack of concern. The inpatient staff must keep in mind that suicide attempters are 140 times more likely to commit suicide than nonattempters and that roughly 10–20 percent of all suicide attempters eventually kill themselves" (pp. 359–360).

Impulsivity and temper tantrums. Temper outbursts, even when not directed at staff, can create feelings of incompetence and helplessness. Patients can often use this gesture effectively as a means of control or to register anger at staff without having to make any direct demands. It is impossible to define all of the possible sources of temper outbursts or violence as there are several factors that may play an important role in this behavior. However, the inability to tolerate affect (such as depression, anxiety, or fear) and a limited ability to formulate a nonviolent response may each play a significant role in this behavior. Common feelings that impulsive behavior can engender in the treater include anger, feelings of revulsion, and fear. When the impulsivity is displayed as blatant violence, these feelings are often more easily recognized and confronted. However, when the event is more insidious, the treater may be in danger of not recognizing the reactions this behavior has aroused:

> Each therapist has personal limits regarding how much anger is tolerable. If the therapist closely monitors counter transference feelings, this limit can be handled constructively rather than destructively. [Gabbard, 1990, p. 356].

Demanding behavior. Demanding patients have always been difficult to treat for staff. These patients disrupt the regular routine by demanding immediate attention to their problems. They cause resentment among other patients because of special attention they may receive. Because no one can ever satisfy their demands, they cause significant counteractions in the staff. Staff feel helpless, frustrated, and even unconsciously incompetent. This may lead treaters to react with anger or, worse, passive-aggressiveness. These patients can threaten staff indirectly by threatening to "reveal" staff incompetence. In fact, in the hospital where I am medical director, some disruptive patients have used the "care connection" phone, a phone line on which patients can register any complaint directly to administration, successfully to that end.

Recognizing the Disruptive Patient

In today's cost-conscious environment, when there are few extra resources available, the system can be stressed more quickly than was once the case. Patients exhibiting disruptive behaviors can, therefore, be especially troublesome. Additionally, as workloads are increasing, the time clinicians have available to work through the myriad issues of countertransference these patients engender is likely diminished and clinicians' ability to launch an effective response hindered. It is, therefore, especially important that the disruptive patient be recognized quickly and dealt with immediately.

Although some patients belonging to difficult populations are easy to identify because of their diagnoses (for example, borderline personality disorder) or their behaviors (for example, suicidal threats), others are less easily identified. When it is not obvious that the team is dealing with a disruptive patient, because the disruptions are below the threshold of obvious detection, counterproductive reactions toward the difficult patient and/or other patients or staff members, can develop. A recent example illustrates this phenomenon (the names used are pseudonyms):

Recently Bill, a young man of seventeen, was admitted to my hospital. Bill was diagnosed with major depression; however, his behavior fit the definition of a disruptive patient, and he likely had a comorbid conduct disorder that was not identified as such early on. Shortly after Bill's admission, Frank was admitted. Frank was diagnosed with an unusual anxiety and impulse disorder. His behavior was obviously disruptive, especially in groups; however, he was neither dangerous nor violent. Bill attempted to convince the staff that Frank's disruptions were provocative and would cause Bill or one of the other patients to lose physical control. The staff were rightly alarmed. However, only Bill's actions were identified as disruptive; the psychiatrist was pressured to take action that led to Bill's eventual transfer. This example involved several well-trained staff members who were all familiar with the concept of countertransference and the potentially manipulative behaviors of many psychiatric patients. However, it was not until after the event occurred that staff were able to identify the role they played in the incident and the way in which Frank manipulated the situation. Unfortunately, these types of incidents brew slowly, creeping up and distorting staff perceptions. Proper identification of disruptive patients early on could have avoided the situation described above.

A second case example involves two middle-aged women with borderline personality disorders on the same unit. On admission, each of them had been given a serious Axis I disorder diagnosis that explained their mood instability. Neither carried the diagnosis of borderline personality disorder. Through the processes of splitting and projective identification, one of the two women developed the "good" personality and the other developed the "bad" and "difficult" personality. The second, "bad" patient was soon viewed as a difficult and ungrateful patient who jeopardized the milieu and perhaps was not appropriate for the unit. In this case, the problem was discovered quickly. Debriefing of the staff brought out the severe countertransference that had developed. A therapeutic protocol was enacted and both women had successful hospitalizations.

How can we identify such patients early? By holding supervision meetings with therapists and other staff in which countertransference issues are discussed, we can minimize these disruptive incidents. Additionally, a thorough evaluation upon admission of personality features, history of family relationships, and disruptions in other intimate personal relationships can help alert the treatment team to the myriad of issues with which the patient may present and can allow the therapist to better formulate an explanation for subsequent disruptive behaviors. This, in turn, can have a positive impact on the management of any disruptive incidents.

Treating and Managing the Disruptive Patient

It is important to understand that not all disruptive patients are psychiatrically ill, nor are all psychiatrically ill patients disruptive. However, many disruptive individuals do have a psychiatric disorder that will respond to treatment. It is often difficult to bear in mind the fact that the disruptive individual is, in fact, suffering from a psychiatric disorder, and despite the difficulty he or she poses, needs and deserves treatment.

It is also important to mention briefly the differentiation between disruptive behaviors and a diagnosis of antisocial personality disorder. Although the research supports the belief that the true antisocial personality disordered patient does not benefit from treatment, this diagnosis is often applied too liberally. Similarly, the diagnosis of conduct disorder is often taken to construe a younger version of the antisocial personality disorder, and the treatability of these patients is similarly discredited. Mislabeling disruptive patients as antisocial does a great disservice to these patients, who in fact, can benefit greatly from treatment.

In addition to requiring treatment and benefiting from it, many disruptive patients also require management if they are to benefit from the psychiatric intervention. Management is distinct from treatment in that some interventions may not aim to produce a distinctly positive therapeutic effect but, instead, to diminish the potential for negative disruptive behaviors. (As the management and treatment of some of the disruptive behaviors commonly seen in borderline patients are addressed in the following section, readers can assume that similar strategies apply to individuals in other diagnostic categories. However, the medication treatments detailed relate specifically to individuals with a diagnosis of BPD. The reader is therefore referred to other literature for psychopharmacological recommendations for other disruptive patients.)

Psychotherapeutic Strategies. Suicidal threats and gestures are the first issue that must be addressed with most borderline patients. Very often the only way to assure their safety is to hospitalize them. One of the key goals of an inpatient hospitalization is to assure that the patient is able to remain safe. The following treatment strategies can help the clinician realize this goal:

- Place the patient on very frequent checks (usually at least every fifteen minutes) as well as suicide precautions. If the patient is even more acute, he or she can be put on line-of-sight or one-to-one supervision. The difference between these latter two precautions is important from a resource utilization standpoint. Line of sight often does not require an extra staff member while one on one almost always does. During day shifts, when there are more staff available and the patients are supposed to be up in the dayroom, line of sight will be adequate for all but the imminently suicidal. At night, one on one will usually be necessary.
- Early in the hospitalization, it is important to begin making the patient responsible for his or her own safety. This is always a difficult step. Taking this step too early could compromise the patient's safety. However not taking this step soon enough could foster the patient's pathological dependencies, which often prove to be at least as much of a risk to the patient's safety. Managing their own safety is one of the most valuable lessons patients can learn. This goal is, of course, long term and will not be fully accomplished on discharge. Helping patients understand how to use the hospital for their safety is an essential short-term goal that should be achieved before discharge.

Unreasonable demandingness is probably the most difficult behavior for staff to handle. In training staff, it is important to see that they understand that some of the difficult patients' demands may be reasonable. I have seen some staff disregard reasonable demands not only from difficult patients but also from other patients, as they assume that all demands from patients are unreasonable. In many ways, demanding behavior is desirable. It is a far more reasonable method of attention seeking than suicidal threats or temper outbursts.

Often the patient does not know how he or she is being perceived by the staff. The patient assumes that he or she is viewed as "low" and disliked and will not receive any attention unless he or she "attacks" with demands. When staff then react with anger at the way they are approached, this only reinforces the patient's perception of low self-esteem. Therefore, it is important for such patients to understand how they affect other human beings. To this end, it is important to instruct staff on how to appropriately share the way these patients make them feel. In conveying these feelings to a patient, staff must be careful not to discuss the patient's behaviors in a critical manner. They must also be very careful when examining their feelings. Often, the first feeling they will find is anger. However, I have found that this is usually not a "true" feeling but rather a projective identification: "All forms of manipulation, persuasion, ingratiating or seduction involve projective identification in the sense that the subject wishes to control an object via influence and subterfuge which, at bottom, involve fantasies of entering into the body of the object in order to effect this control" (Grotstein, 1985, pp. 180–181). Thus, when staff members carefully examine their feelings in such cases, they find that helplessness, doubt, and despair often are underneath. Thus, they might say to the patient, "When you talk to me this way, I feel that I have offended you and not done my job. I feel helpless to meet your needs and that makes me sad." If this sounds contrived, I suggest that is because we defend against such feelings with great might.

The key to mitigating the negative impact of a patient's projective identification is the ability of the staff to address how various behaviors make them feel. Therefore, the patient is introduced to feedback on the effects of his or her behavior on other human beings. Although this may seem to be a very simple point which we learn in "Therapy 101," we do not often systematically apply it on an organizational level. Furthermore, I rarely see it reflected in treatment plans, nor do I hear it discussed in treatment teams. This strategy is likely to be considerably more difficult to apply with narcissistic patients who are more heavily defended. However, achieving this kind of honest relationship with borderline patients not only helps in defusing unreasonable demands but also helps to defuse temper outbursts, projection defenses, and suicidal threats.

The next step is to encourage the patient to become responsible to others. This is often attempted in a dry and personally meaningless way and therefore fails. Again, the key is the ability to share one's emotions in a therapeutic fashion. Once patients understand the negative effect their behavior has on others, they should become aware of how to have the opposite effect. To this end, a patient may begin to ask not for services but for more feedback, until he or she can model behaviors which make his or her company more desirable. I mention this advanced strategy because hospital staffs will encounter borderline patients at all levels of recovery and because these patients can become suicidal at any level of recovery. However, most patient-staff encounters are likely not to be up to these advanced strategies.

Pharmacological Management. The psychiatrist should carefully consider the medication strategy, with the immediate postdischarge period in mind. Many difficult patients will still have a degree of suicidality when released and for many months afterward. Anticipating this, selective serotonin reoptake inhibitors (SSRIs) and Trazodone, which have lower suicide potential than TCAs, should be used when possible. An exception to this use might be fluoxetine. Although fluoxetine is a very good medication, one must anticipate that at some time in the future, if the patient should have a medication failure, a monoamine oxidase inhibitor (MAOI) may become appropriate. Because fluoxetine's required washout period is five weeks, this could leave the patient psychopharmacologically uncovered for too long.

In deciding whether to prescribe an MAOI to a borderline patient, I evaluate the impulsiveness of the patient. If the impulsiveness is low enough and other antidepressants have failed, a well-watched MAOI trial may be in order. In these cases, I usually prefer to hospitalize the patient for such a trial. The psychiatric hospital milieu is very effective in reducing impulsive behavior. Diet can be well controlled and emergency personnel are at hand. Doses can be titrated much more quickly as well. If the MAOI has the desired response, then impulsiveness will decrease radically and the patient is then as safe as most other patients on MAOIs (Dunner, 1993).

Next to the antidepressants, I find low-dose neuroleptics very valuable in controlling the borderline patient's disruptive behaviors. Patients feel so much better on these medications, usually in forty-eight hours, that they are reluctant to give them up some months later to evaluate their ability to go without them. The benefit of the neuroleptic must be weighed against the higher-than-average risk these patients may have for tardive dyskinesia (TD). Often, however, one to two milligrams of Navane, or its equivalent, will be extremely effective. If five milligrams (or equivalent) of Navane is not effective, the patient is not likely to respond to neuroleptics and higher doses are usually not worth the risk, since TD is also dose dependent (Dunner, 1993).

Although Tegretol has been shown to be useful when it works, it generally does so only after about a month. Therefore, it is not useful in the most acute phase. It is important that when the patients leave the confines of the hospital, which are so effective in controlling suicidality and impulsiveness, that they have tools to protect them. Without rapidly effective medications, they leave the hospital without the full protection of the medication (Dunner, 1993).

Finally, I should note that one must be very careful in the use of benzodiazepines in these patients. Borderline patients in general should not receive benzodiazepines. Their disruptive and dangerous behaviors can become significantly worse. Furthermore, the interpersonal lessons discussed above, when learned under the influence of the benzodiazepines, may not be generalizable. Having said this, there may be a few cases in which borderline patients have comorbid panic attacks or chronic insomnia that benzodiazepines may be useful. However, I would be careful to avoid such drugs until the patient has been stabilized on other medications to minimize the risk of emotional dyscontrol. I especially recommend the same cautions for patients with multiple personality disorder (Dunner, 1993).

Conclusion

Crisis stabilization alone is often not a sufficient goal for BPD patients. The overall costs of not addressing the chronicity and recurrence of the borderline patient's problems in the long run will be higher morbidity and higher costs, through readmission and treatment failures. At the same time, one cannot attempt to address all of the patient's problems in one hospitalization. Rather an integrated treatment plan must be laid out, which uses different levels of care to address the entire illness. When a reputable payer can be given a sensible treatment plan, incorporating all of the important factors, the payer can attempt to match resources needed. Furthermore, progress toward the goals can be monitored.

To successfully treat difficult-to-treat patients and handle their disruptive behavior, a hospital must engage the entire treatment team and the administration as well. The team must first have a good communication system. Without this, patients' projective identifications will cause severe splitting. The team members must also learn to identify countertransferences in themselves and co-workers. They must act as supports for each other, helping each other to be truly honest with his or her feelings. Staff members can productively encourage each other to learn and assure each person of his or her competence, lest there be a weakness that can be exploited. In communicating with the psychiatrist, staff must be able to understand what he or she wishes to accomplish with psychopharmacology, so that they can properly report back on progress. They must understand what the therapist's goals are as well.

Administration can help in the treatment of the difficult patient by making training time available. At one of the hospitals where I have attended, one of the service directors developed a weekly training session he called "countertransference rounds." Currently at Canyon Springs Hospital, we have weekly training sessions that deal with such countertransference issues. We also teach technical skills and perform "rehearsals" of therapeutic situations, so that when confronted by disruptive behaviors, our staff will be familiar with the situation. Administration can also be useful by supporting continuous quality improvement projects that examine efficacy of treatment of these behaviors. These can always be classified as problem-prone issues, often as high-risk issues, and sometimes even as high-volume issues.

The experience of working with disruptive patients does not have to be negative. In fact, with appropriate application of the strategies and techniques discussed above, the disruptive behaviors can be effectively mitigated and the overall experience can become a positive challenge for the treatment team.

References

Dunner, D. L. *Current Psychiatric Therapy*. London: W. B. Saunders, 1993.

Gabbard, G. O. *Psychodynamic Psychiatry in Clinical Practice*. Washington, D.C., 1990.

Grotstein, J. S. *Splitting and Projective Identification*. Northvale, N.J.: Jason Aronson, Inc., 1985.

Gunderson, J. G. *Borderline Personality Disorder*. Washington, D.C.: American Psychiatric Press, 1984.

Roth, S. *Psychotherapy: The Art of Wooing Nature*. Northvale, N.J.: Jason Aronson, 1987.

Widiger, T. A., and Frances, A. J. "Epidemiology, Diagnosis, and Comorbidity of Borderline Personality Disorder." *American Psychiatric Press Review of Psychiatry*, 1989, *8*.

LES ALHADEFF, M.D., is medical director of Canyon Springs Hospital.

PART THREE

Non-Clinical Challenges in an Inpatient Setting

Developments in outcomes research and assessment of value in psychiatric hospital treatment reveal that outcomes measurement fits into an overall assessment of value, works with multidimensional outcomes, and has practical applications that enhance the quality of psychiatric services.

The Assessment of Outcome and Value of Psychiatric Hospital Treatment

Stephen F. Butler, John P. Docherty

Interest in assessing outcomes of treatment for both medical-surgical and psychiatric treatment has virtually exploded over the last few years. This development has paralleled a radical change in the primary goals and objectives, mission, and expectations of health care in this country. The last three decades were devoted to a strong central national concern with the development of new, demonstrably effective treatments. Institutions such as the National Institutes of Health and many other governmental initiatives were established to support this work. The focus of medical research during this era was on clinical trials, whose objective was to determine the safety and efficacy of precisely defined treatments under highly controlled conditions. The health care field was remarkably successful in accomplishing this mission.

Recently, however, the realization of these successes has been accompanied by an increasing sense of crisis in health care delivery. This crisis has been fueled by staggering increases in costs of health care over the last three decades. Health care costs have risen from $50 billion in 1960 to $90 billion in 1973 to $500 billion (11 percent of the gross national product) in 1986 (Zimet, 1989) to $735 billion in 1991 (Resnick, 1992). These dramatic cost increases have resulted in changes in the mission with which the health care field is charged. The new mission tasks the health care field with moving beyond treatment developments to enhance the care of the individual patient and to develop methods and procedures to advance the well-being of the entire collectivity.

Rather than being questions about the safety and efficacy of experimental treatments, the essential questions for outcomes research are real-world ones of effectiveness: What outcomes are actually achieved, for which patients, and at what cost? Or, more succinctly put, What is the value of the treatment in question? The answers to these questions are expected to have practical utility in improving health care quality. This chapter addresses the broad developments in the area of outcomes research and assessment of value in psychiatric hospital treatment. It also discusses the practical application of these developments to enhance the quality of psychiatric services.

The use of the word *value* reflects a momentous shift of perspective for all medicine, including psychiatry. Valuable mental health service is service that yields *good* outcomes *efficiently* (Docherty and Butler, 1993). This means that acceptable effectiveness is achieved as quickly as possible, in the least restrictive setting possible, with patients matched to appropriate treatments and levels of care.

Thus, the concept of value encompasses the ultimate goal to which policymakers, providers, patients, and payers aspire: namely, a level of efficiency that serves to control costs while yielding acceptable outcomes. This goal, in turn, implies the ability to track costs, to measure administrative and clinical processes, to measure patient outcomes and satisfaction, and to integrate these data (costs, processes, and outcomes) in a way that enhances policy and clinical decision making. Thus, embedded in the concept of value for mental health services is the need for a comprehensive system that permits statistical analysis of outcomes and processes. Until recently, analysis of outcomes data relied heavily on case review, which tends to be time consuming, labor intensive, and of limited utility in addressing broad-based questions of quality (Goldfield, Pine, and Pine, 1992). The advent of computer technology, however, renders possible patient tracking, data collection and storage, and analysis that is carried out on a large scale and within a reasonable time frame. This ability to collect, analyze, and provide virtually instantaneous feedback to providers, payers, and other interested parties, makes possible a real revolution in the practical use of outcomes data. Presently, as the Jackson Hole Group notes, in general, clinicians "do not have access to an information base from which . . . responsible, informed choices can be made" (Ellwood, Etheredge, and the Jackson Hole Group, 1991, p. 1). However, these authors go on to note that in a "21st century health system . . . each provider group must be held publicly accountable for the impact (in terms of cost, effectiveness, and patient values) of the care they deliver" (p. 2).

Reliable outcome data, therefore, are increasingly being recognized as an essential first step in making treatment decisions that incorporate advances in the scientific understanding of the etiology and treatment of psychiatric disorders (Mirin and Namerow, 1991). In fact, market pressure from payers and patients, coupled with mandates from regulatory agencies such as the Joint Commission on Accreditation of Healthcare Organizations (JCAHO), are rapidly causing outcomes measurement to become obligatory.

Outcomes Research in Psychiatry

In this section, we discuss central issues involved in the conceptualization, development, and implementation of a system for enhancing the value of psychiatric services.

Determining the Value of Psychiatric Services. Table 7.1 presents a schematic diagram of the main components of a comprehensive value accounting system for psychiatric services (Docherty and Butler, 1993). The system consists of two main components. One is a traditional system for fiscal accounting, that is, a system which provides a detailed quantitative account and analysis of the costs of providing service. The second component is a quantitative quality accounting system. It is a given that a financial accounting system is necessary and useful to a successful business. The concept of value accounting extends this procedure to quality. As in fiscal accounting, where managers can track how an organization is doing financially, a quality accounting system quantifies key facets of quality to yield a similar tracking capability. Thus, quality and fiscal measures are conceptualized as parallel contributors to the overall value of services provided.

The conceptualization illustrated in Table 7.1 derives from a classic health services research paradigm for evaluation (for example, Kiesler, Simpkins, and

Table 7.1. Value Accounting System for Psychiatric Services

		Value Components	*Measurement Domains*	*Indicator Categories*	*Assessment Tools*
VALUE	*Quality Accounting*	*Service*	Resources and personnel	Suitable Sufficient Aesthetic	Credentialing Staffing guidelines Patient characteristics
			Clinical and administrative procedures and processes	Appropriate Necessary Current Competent Compassionate	Practice guidelines Critical incidents Quality audits
		Effectiveness	Outcomes	Access Satisfaction Clinical effectiveness	Patient satisfaction GAF SF-36 Self-report (symptom, functioning, well-being)
	Fiscal Accounting	*Cost*	Cost	Cost Cost-benefit Cost effectiveness	Cost of resources and personnel Treatment utilization Cost-offset

Morton, 1991; Newman and Sorensen, 1988), and it assumes that an acceptable quality accounting system should provide quantitative measurement of the quality of key dimensions in three domains: the resources and personnel used to provide service; the actual clinical and administrative procedures constituting and supporting the provision of service; and the effectiveness of service, including consumer (patient, payer) satisfaction and clinical outcome, measuring separately symptoms, social function, work function, and treatment utilization. A fourth domain contains fiscal data, that is, the assessment of cost. Relevant characteristics of each domain are listed, as are some possible ways to quantify (that is, operationalize) the dimension.[1]

The calculation of value then becomes a conceptually simple procedure. Value is the intersection between the cost (or price) of a service and the quality of that service. As Table 7.1 illustrates, the measurement of value is achieved by the marriage of a quality accounting system and a fiscal accounting system. Implementation of some of the important aspects of such a system are described below; however, we first turn to the general issue of operationally defining the basic independent and dependent variables.

Definition of Key Variables. There are two key variables: outcome, a dependent variable, and treatment, an independent variable.

Outcome: the dependent variable. Like any other research, outcomes research requires that the dependent and independent variables be defined and operationalized. The dependent variable for outcomes research is outcome itself. While at first glance this may seem self-evident, a precise definition of mental health outcome can be quite difficult to pin down. Outcomes in medical-surgical specialties may be more easily defined. Mortality rates, for instance, or presence versus absence of infection provide relatively unambiguous measures of outcome.[2] However, more sophisticated views of outcome, including medical-surgical outcomes, are moving beyond simple resolution of an acute episode of a disorder. Rather, outcome now refers to the "extent to which a change in the patient's functioning or well-being meets the patient's needs or expectations" (Ware, 1993). In this sense, outcome is clearly a multidimensional construct, consisting not only of changes in symptomatology or psychiatric functioning, but of patient satisfaction, treatment utilization rates, and social and work functioning as well.

A further consideration in psychiatric outcome reflects the notion that outcome can be viewed from different perspectives that are related but not identical (Strupp and Hadley, 1977). For any particular patient, there are at least three perspectives on patient outcome, represented by the following stakeholders: the clinician, the patient, and society (which may include the patient's family, employer, third-party payer, and so forth). Each of these perspectives reflects different values. For example, the clinician may be most interested in the clinical status of the patient, including for instance, reduction in suicidality, improvement in specific symptomatology, and reduction in substance use. The patient may value most return to family, improvement in general distress level, and so forth. Finally, the employer is interested in the patient's ability to function at work, the third-party payer is interested in reduced utilization of medical services, and the community is interested in reduced utilization of criminal justice resources. The patient's family, too, may have a unique perspective on the kind of outcome desired. Any outcome-based quality evaluation must take into account at least some of these different perspectives.

Treatment: the independent variable. Defining and measuring the treatment in an outcome study presents as many difficulties as defining and measuring outcome. Recognition in the 1970s that different psychotherapists, even those who profess the same theoretical orientation, actually conduct therapy quite differently led to the development of psychotherapy "manuals" in an effort to standardize the delivery of treatments in clinical trial research (Butler and Strupp, 1993). It is rarely the case that such precision is possible in outcomes research—particularly with inpatient treatment consisting of a variety of different groups and therapies, as well as more informal contacts with staff.

In our experience, it is practical and useful to characterize treatment more broadly. We recommend the inclusion of such variables as the setting (inpatient versus partial hospital versus outpatient), the particular unit or treatment team, the attending or other provider, and the types and amounts of services rendered (length of stay, type and amount of group therapy, type and amount of individual therapy, use of psychopharmacological agents, and so forth). Clearly, greater specificity of treatments provided permits more precise questions to be addressed. Nevertheless, much can be learned from examining the outcomes of treatments in this more broadly defined way. It is particularly useful to follow trends over time and compare attending clinicians and treatment teams to each other and to clinical benchmarks (described later). Such procedures can give clinical managers vital information on which to base clinical decisions.

Outcomes Research Implementation

The following discussion reflects adherence to the following principles: the measures selected to evaluate outcomes should be comprehensive in scope, cost-effective to use, impose minimal burden on staff and patients, and have evidence of adequate reliability and validity.

Clinician Ratings. The perspective of the treating clinician can be obtained using the Global Assessment of Functioning (GAF) scale. The GAF provides a summary score of the patient's overall health status. This includes an assessment of the symptom picture, but the focus of the GAF also captures the impact of symptoms on the patient's social and occupational functioning. Thus, the presence of a symptom like hearing voices is rated, but the schizophrenic who is currently too disorganized or suicidal to function without supervision is rated much lower than one who is able to maintain a daily routine.

Global scales, like the GAF, are relatively easy to use in that they do not require special interviews or inordinate clinician time, and they are inexpensive to process and analyze. Global scales have good face validity and integrate multidimensional decisions made about patients (Newman, 1980). Global ratings have been shown to maintain reliability and validity when they are used routinely in clinical settings and when staff are regularly trained in the proper use of the scale (Newman, 1980). Finally, the GAF is widely used and recognized by the agencies and institutions interested in outcome assessment.

Potential limitations to using the GAF are the same ones that could be leveled against all psychiatric global ratings: that such scales yield only a coarse measure of patient status or that they are subjective and, as such, invalid. However, measures of overall severity, like the GAF, have the distinct advantage of summarizing many elements of psychopathology into a single, clinically meaningful index of severity of illness (Endicott, Spitzer, Fleiss, and Cohen, 1976). Furthermore, the evidence does not support the contention that such scales are invalid. Global ratings of patient status tend to be more sensitive to differential treatment effects than, for instance, measures of single dimensions of psychopathology (see, for example, McGlashan, 1973). The predecessor of the GAF, the Global Assessment Scale (GAS), correlates with psychosis/neurosis diagnoses, recidivism, use of mental health resources, and in-depth (that is, interview) measures of adjustment (Newman, 1980). The GAF is widely used in outcome research and, with training, yields reliable and valid ratings of patient functioning.

In order to establish and monitor inter-rater reliability on GAF ratings, a training program should be instituted. A GAF training program has been developed using standard clinical vignettes (Endicott, 1991), and this program is described in greater detail elsewhere (Docherty and Butler, 1993). Comparisons of pre- and posttraining GAF ratings suggest that the training is effective in improving inter-rater reliability.

Patient Ratings. As previously described, outcome is a complex multidimensional construct comprised of semi-independent dimensions of symptomatology, social and work function, and satisfaction with treatment and health care resource utilization. An evaluation system should specifically address each of these issues.

Symptomatology. Obviously, symptoms are an important dimension of outcome. Symptoms constitute the basis of diagnostic considerations and are critical to treatment planning. Furthermore, in most cases, some form of symptomatic distress is involved in the patient's seeking psychiatric treatment. Finally, improvement in this area is expected by the stakeholders (clinicians, patients, families, and so forth). There are a number of easy-to-use symptom checklists. Examples include the Symptom Checklist-90-R (Derogatis, 1977) or its shorter version, the Brief Symptom Inventory (BSI) (Derogatis and Melisaratos, 1983). Another example is the Basis-32 developed by Eisen and colleagues at McLean's Hospital (Eisen, Grob, and Klein, 1986).

Functioning. The patient's ability to function in social and occupational roles is increasingly recognized as a critical outcome dimension, on a par with symptomatic concerns. Particularly with chronic disabilities, which include many psychiatric and substance abuse disorders, a major impact of treatment may be on the patient's ability to resume role responsibilities. Also, as previously described, functioning is of particular concern to employers, third-party payers, and other community interests. The SF-36 Health Status Survey (Ware and Sherbourne, 1992; Ware, Snow, Kosinski, and Gandek, 1993), which was developed as part of the RAND Corporation's Medical Outcomes Study (MOS), is a particularly useful instrument for this domain.

Client satisfaction. An additional part of the domain of effectiveness reflects the degree to which the interventions have met the expectations and needs of the patients. When assessing improvement achieved through medical interventions, attention must be paid to this area (Ware, 1993). Probably the most widely recognized existing scale for assessing patient satisfaction is the Client Satisfaction Questionnaire (CSQ) developed by Attkisson and Associates (Larsen, Attkisson, Hargraves, and Nguyen, 1979; Nguyen, Attkisson, and Stegner, 1983). This eight-item questionnaire has been used in several published accounts of evaluations of mental health programs, and these different accounts provide some basis of comparison (see, for example, Nguyen, Attkisson, and Stegner, 1983; Sishta, Rinco, and Sullivan, 1986). It may be desirable to add to the CSQ items that address directly areas of concern to the particular facility.

Collection of satisfaction data presents several dilemmas. The appropriate use of patient satisfaction data is to focus on those instances where clients have indicated some level of dissatisfaction (Larsen, Attkisson, Hargraves, and Nguyen, 1979). Areas of service with which patients express dissatisfaction should be targeted for further examination, according to continuous quality improvement principles. Thus, it is critical for patients to feel free to indicate dissatisfaction, and in general, it is important to avoid procedures that might discourage patients from expressing dissatisfaction. For example, patients may feel encouraged to speak freely when outside consulting firms are used to survey the patients after discharge or termination from treatment. However, contacting patients by mail after they leave often results in poor response rates, which can limit the utility of the satisfaction data. Telephone interviews two or three weeks after discharge or termination are likely to improve the response rate. By implementing safeguards that obviously protect specific patient identities, procedures can also be developed for effective collection of satisfaction data in-house.

There may be no clearly criticism-proof methodology for collecting satisfaction data. The best strategy, as with any research, is to delineate clearly the use to which the data are to be put (for example, staff feedback versus marketing). This strategy makes it more likely that the procedures designed will achieve particular goals within budgetary constraints.

Resource utilization. Another important outcome that can be assessed with self-reporting is the effectiveness of medical resources used by the patient. Third-party payers and employers are often interested in whether expensive interventions such as psychiatric hospitalization result in a decrease in utilization of subsequent medical procedures. Patients can be asked at intake or on admission about their utilization of medical treatments and this report can be compared to answers given at follow-up. Since improved psychological functioning is likely to affect general health (Schlesinger and Mumford, 1984; Wells and others, 1989), it is important to ask about medical-surgical hospitalizations, emergency room visits, and visits to physicians for medical problems, along with utilization of services for emotional or substance abuse problems.

Assessment of an intervention's impact on medical resource utilization has traditionally been accomplished using insurance company data bases. Using patient self-reports to estimate resource utilization is a relatively new area of research. Probably the best known instrument is an interview called the Treatment Services Review (TSR) developed by McLellan (McLellan and others, 1992). The use of special interviews, while appropriate for specialized studies, is of less practical utility for ongoing assessments of large numbers of patients.

Follow-up. Follow-up data are essential to gain a complete picture of the benefit gained as the result of an intervention. For inpatients, the dimensions of outcome reflecting functioning are truly meaningful only after discharge. While symptom improvement and global distress may be reliably assessed at discharge, it takes time outside the hospital to determine whether or not the patient returns to premorbid levels of functioning. It is also important to know the extent of relapse for particular categories of patients.

An initial step is to establish a time frame for the follow-up. Often, it is useful to obtain follow-up at two points: one reflecting a short lapse of time and presumably more directly influenced by the index hospitalization, and one reflecting a longer lapse of time. Information about the expected course of particular disorders can be helpful in selecting an appropriate time frame. Depression, for instance, is a common diagnostic category in psychiatric hospitals. For this group, a follow-up assessment at six months would reflect a time frame long enough to detect patients' response to treatment (Keller and others, 1992) and a follow-up at twelve months should cover a long enough period to capture relapse (Shea and others, 1992; Frank and others, 1990). Similar time frames would likely be appropriate for substance abuse diagnoses.

In addition, additional background and demographic information can greatly enhance the value of the clinical data and expand the analyses that can be conducted with that data. We recommend that data on the variables outlined in the following paragraphs be collected. (These variables are consistent with guidelines published by the NIMH for essential clinical management data.)

Identifying variables. It is necessary to uniquely identify a treatment episode for each particular patient. There are typically three variables required to uniquely identify a treatment episode: the *medical record number,* a *facility or program number,* and an *episode number.*

Patient demographics. It is essential to describe who the patient is. Variables such as age, sex, marital status, origin, and zip code are necessary to adequately describe the population of patients to whom treatment is being given.

Patient diagnosis. Just like demographics, comprehensive chart diagnoses are essential. They must include the primary diagnosis along with all diagnoses on all axes. These diagnoses should be entered according to their DSM-III-R (or DSM-IV) diagnostic code, since numeric data is more easily manipulated.

Dates of treatment. For inpatients, this variable refers to admission and discharge dates. From these data, length of stay can be calculated and readmission (recidivism) can be tracked. For patients in partial hospital or intensive outpatient programs, we recommend gathering both the dates of inclusion in the program and the number of hours per week the patient participates. This helps differentiate the patient seen fifteen hours per week for five weeks from the patient seen five hours per week for fifteen weeks.

Payer information. Information should be obtained that identifies the primary guarantor. The codes for these data permit the classification of patients into payer categories. Information about secondary guarantors should also be recorded.

Primary provider/attending. For inpatients this is usually a physician or psychologist. Each attending clinician should have a unique identification code.

Service identifiers. The most basic treatment descriptor is a service code, which identifies the patient as either an inpatient, partial hospital, or outpatient. Other categorizations can be determined as appropriate to the facility or system being evaluated.

Program or unit identifiers. The next level of treatment descriptor is a program and/or unit code. Sometimes both program and unit codes are needed to clearly identify the treatment program for a given patient. For instance, a unit number may reveal that a patient was on an adult unit while the program number may show that the patient was in a dual diagnosis track or program on that unit.

Treatment components. Treatment elements can be more specifically coded and entered in order to describe the presence of pharmacological treatment, amount and type of group therapies, vocational or other counseling, amount and type of individual therapy services, and so forth.

Conclusion

Clinicians are entering a revolutionary era in which outcomes research will become an intrinsic aspect of psychiatric care. While compliance with the regulations of JCAHO and other accrediting agencies along with demands of payers to demonstrate effectiveness may drive this revolution, the ultimate goal of outcomes measurement and management is to achieve a higher-quality outcome (product or service). Viewed in this way, the specific recent impetus for measuring and managing mental health outcome has at its core questions of vital interest to the practice of psychiatry. There are fundamental questions about the treatment of mental disorders for which psychiatry has no clear answers. Such questions include asking about the appropriate treatments, settings, providers, and/or levels or intensity of care for patients with particular diagnoses or sets of problems. The evidence suggests there is substantial diversity of opinion on the treatment of choice for any particular psychiatric disorder (American Psychiatric Association Commission on Psychiatric Therapies, 1982, 1984a, 1984b). As desirable outcomes are identified and agreed upon, practice patterns will become more consistent. Demonstrably unnecessary or ineffective approaches to treatments will be abandoned, while those yielding superior outcomes at reasonable costs will find greater application.

Notes

1. A description of procedures for evaluating administrative procedures and establishing costs is beyond the scope of this chapter. Interested readers are referred to Docherty and Butler (1993) for further information regarding these domains.
2. It is easy to become discouraged at the "softness" of psychiatric measures of outcome. However, in our opinion, such discouragement is unwarranted. Many seemingly objective measures of medical outcomes have undergone less rigorous reliability and validity testing than measures of psychiatric outcome (see, for example, Newman, 1980).

References

American Psychiatric Association Commission on Psychiatric Therapies. *Psychotherapy Research: Methodological and Efficacy Issues.* Washington, D.C.: American Psychiatric Association, 1982.

American Psychiatric Association Commission on Psychiatric Therapies. Vol. 1: *The Psychiatric Therapies.* Washington, D.C.: American Psychiatric Association, 1984a.

American Psychiatric Association Commission on Psychiatric Therapies. Vol. 1: *The Psychiatric Therapies.* Washington, D.C.: American Psychiatric Association 1984b.

Butler, S. F., and Strupp, H. H. "The Effects of Training Psychoanalytically Oriented Therapists to Use a Manual." In N. E. Miller, L. Luborsky, J. P. Barber, and J. Docherty (eds.), *Handbook of Dynamic Psychotherapy: Research and Practice.* New York: Basic Books, 1993.

Deming, W. E. *Out of the Crisis.* Cambridge: Massachusetts Institute of Technology, Center for Advanced Engineering Study, 1986.

Derogatis, L. R. *SCL-90: Administration, Scoring, and Procedures Manual for the Revised Version.* 1977. (Available from the author, Adolf Meyer Building, Room 200, The Johns Hopkins Hospital, 600 N. Wolfe St., Baltimore, MD 21205.

Derogatis, L. R., and Melisaratos, N. "The Brief Symptom Inventory: An Introductory Report." *Psychological Medicine,* 1983, *13,* 595–605.

Docherty, J. P., and Butler, S. F. "A Comprehensive System for Value Accounting in Psychiatry." Manuscript submitted for publication, 1993.

Eisen, S. V., Grob, M. C., and Klein, A. A. "Basis: The Development of a Self-Report Measure for Psychiatric Inpatient Evaluation." *The Psychiatric Hospital,* 1986, *17,* 165–171.

Ellwood, P., Etheredge, L., and the Jackson Hole Group. *Overview and Accountable Health Partnerships: The 2lst Century American Health System.* Policy Doc. no. 1 of 4. Teton Village, Wyo.: The Jackson Hole Group, 1991.

Endicott, J. *GAF Vignettes.* New York: Department of Research Assessment and Treatment, New York State Psychiatric Institute, 1991.

Endicott, J., Spitzer, R. L., Fleiss, J. L., and Cohen J. "The Global Assessment Scale: A Procedure for Measuring Overall Severity of Psychiatric Disturbance." *Archives of General Psychiatry,* 1976, *33,* 766–771.

Frank, E., Kupfer, D. J., Perel, J. M., Cornes, C., Jarrett, D. B., Mallinger, A. G., Thaje, M. E., McEachron, A. B., and Grochocinski, V. J. "Three Year Outcomes for Maintenance Therapies in Recurrent Depression." *Archives of General Psychiatry,* 1990, *47,* 1093–1099.

Goldfield, N., Pine, M., and Pine, J. *Measuring and Managing Health Care Quality: Procedures, Techniques, and Protocols.* Gaithersburg, Md.: Aspen Publications, 1992.

Joint Commission on Accreditation of Healthcare Organizations. *Transitions: From Qa to Cqi: An Introduction to Quality Improvement in Health Care.* Oakbrook Terrace, Ill.: Joint Commission on Accreditation of Healthcare Organizations, 1991.

Joint Commission on Accreditation of Healthcare Organizations. *The Transition from QA to QI: Performance-Based Evaluation of Mental Health Organizations.* Oakbrook Terrace, Ill.: Joint Commission on Accreditation of Healthcare Organizations, 1992.

Keller, M. B., Lavori, P. W., Mueller, T. I., Endicott, J., Coryell, W., Hirschfeld, R.M.A., and Shea, M. T. "Time to Recovery, Chronicity, and Levels of Psychopathology in Major Depression: A 5-Year Prospective Follow-Up of 431 Subjects." *Archives of General Psychiatry,* 1992, *49,* 809–816.

Kiesler, C. A., Simpkins, C. G., and Morton, T. L. "Research Issues in Mental Health Policy." In M. Hersen, A. E. Kazdin, and A. S. Bellack (eds.), *The Clinical Psychology Handbook* (2nd. ed.). New York, N.Y.: Pergamon Press, 1991.

Larsen, D. L., Attkisson, C. C., Hargraves, W. A., and Nguyen, T. D. "Assessment of Client/Patient Satisfaction: Development of a General Scale." *Evaluation and Program Planning,* 1979, *2,* 197–207.

McGlashan, T. (ed.). *The Documentation of Clinical Psychotropic Drug Trials.* Rockville, Md.: National Institute of Mental Health, 1973.

McLellan, A. T., Alterman, A. I., Cacciola, J., Metzger, D., and O'Brien, C. P. "A New Measure of Substance Abuse Treatment: Initial Studies of the Treatment Services Review." *Journal of Nervous and Mental Disease,* 1992, *180,* 101–110.

Mirin, S. M., and Namerow, M. J. "Why Study Treatment Outcome?" In S. M. Mirin, J. T. Gossett, and M. C. Grob (eds.), *Psychiatric Treatment: Advances in Outcome Research.* Washington, D.C.: American Psychiatric Press, 1991.

Newman, F. L. "Global Scales: Strengths, Uses and Problems of Global Scales as an Evaluation Instrument." *Evaluation and Program Planning,* 1980, *3,* 257–268.

Newman, F. L., and Sorensen, J. E. *Integrated Clinical & Fiscal Management in Mental Health: A Guidebook.* Norwood, N.J.: Ablex, 1988.

Nguyen, T. D., Attkisson, C. C., and Stegner, B. L. "Assessment of Patient Satisfaction: Development and Refinement of a Service Evaluation Questionnaire." *Evaluation and Program Planning,* 1983, *6,* 299–314.

Resnick, R. J. "National Health Is Coming: An Update." *Minnesota Psychologist,* 1992, *41,* 9.

Schlesinger, H. J., and Mumford, E. "The Role of Evidence in the Formulation of Public Policy About Psychotherapy." In J.B.W. Williams and R. L. Spitzer (eds.), *Psychotherapy Research: Where Are We and Where Should We Go?* New York: Guilford Press, 1984.

Shea, M. T., Elkin, I., Imber, S. D., Sotsky, S. M., Watkins, J. T., Collins, J. F., Pilkonis, P. A., Beckham, E., Glass, D. R., Dolan, R. T., and others. "Course of Depressive Symptoms over Follow-Up." Findings from the National Institute of Mental Health Treatment of Depression Collaborative Research Program. *Archives of General Psychiatry,* 1992, *49* (10), 782–787.

Sishta, S. K., Rinco, S., and Sullivan, J.C.F. "Clients' Satisfaction Survey in a Psychiatric Inpatient Population Attached to a General Hospital." *Canadian Journal of Psychiatry,* 1986, *31,* 123–128.

Strupp, H. H., and Hadley, S. W. "A Tripartite Model of Mental Health and Therapeutic Outcomes: With Special Reference to Negative Effects in Psychotherapy." *American Psychologist,* 1977, *32,* 187–196.

Ware, J. E. "Measures for a New Era of Health Assessment." In A. L. Stewart and J. E. Ware (eds.), *Measuring Functioning and Well-Being: The Medical Outcome Study Approach.* Durham, N.C.: Duke University Press, 1993.

Ware, J. E., and Sherbourne, C. D. "The MOS 36-Item Short-Form Health Survey (SF-36): Conceptual Framework and Item Selection." *Medical Care,* 1992, *30,* 473–483.
Ware, J. E., Snow, K. K., Kosinski, M., and Gandek, B. *SF-36 Health Survey: Manual and Interpretation Guide.* Boston: The Health Institute, New England Medical Center, 1993.
Wells, K. B., Stewart, A., Hays, R. D., Burnam, M. A., Rogers, W., Daniels, M., Berry, S., Greenfield, S., and Ware, J. "The Functioning and Well-Being of Depressed Patients: Results from the Medical Outcomes Study." *Journal of the American Medical Association,* 1989, *262,* 914–919.
Zimet, C. N. "The Mental Health Care Revolution: Will Psychology Survive?" *American Psychologist,* 1989, *44,* 703–708.

STEPHEN F. BUTLER, Ph.D., works in the Psychiatric Division of National Medical Enterprises, Inc., and is director of psychology at Nashua Brookside Hospital.

JOHN P. DOCHERTY, M.D., is professor of clinical psychiatry and medical director of the Mental Health Group at the University of California, Los Angeles.

To aid clinicians in preventing adverse legal outcomes, this chapter explains the pressing legal issues currently affecting inpatient psychiatric facilities, including informed consent, liability, and patient rights.

One Axiom and Eight Corollaries for Managing Legal Issues in an Inpatient Psychiatric Setting

Harold J. Bursztajn

Any contemporary textbook on inpatient psychiatry would be incomplete without a substantial section devoted to the legal issues that exert an impact on inpatient clinicians. The past twenty years have spawned a changing but increasingly expanding body of legislation and case law regarding the rights, care, and treatment of the mentally ill. One result of this growth has been an expansion of the contact points between psychiatry and the law, especially in the areas of criminal, victim compensation, and family law. Since numerous books have been written on these classical contact points, I will focus on the emerging areas of contact, where the inpatient psychiatrist's understanding of medicolegal issues is also critical to the care of any hospitalized patient. In particular, the exercise of good judgment and careful understanding of today's most pressing legal issues regarding informed consent, liability, and patient rights is a must if developments around these issues are to enhance rather than compromise the quality of hospitalized patients' care. Therefore, this chapter will focus on integrating emerging legal requirements into the clinical process.

The basic axiom of the following chapter (that is, the fundamental premise on which a successful approach to managing the typical legal issues that arise in an inpatient setting is based) is that informed consent now ought to be used as a *process* rather than *pro forma*, and that informed consent is not

---

This chapter is adapted from H. Bursztajn, T. G. Gutheil, and B. Cummins, "Legal Issues in Inpatient Psychiatry," in L. Sederer (ed.), *Inpatient Psychiatry*, 3rd ed. (Baltimore: Williams & Wilkins, 1991).

only an essential clinical and risk management tool but also an essential tool for helping patients and their families receive the full benefits to which they are entitled.

The eight corollaries to this basic axiom are:

Patients, and where clinically indicated their families, need to be encouraged to become informed of the benefits they are entitled to by contract or state mandate.

Whenever possible, clinician communication with managed care should be not only with the patient's consent but with his or her active participation.

Such communication should be integrated into the patient's treatment program rather than treated as simply "business" or "administration." While those dimensions need to be acknowledged, helping the hospitalized patient relearn how to conduct business or administrate can be an important component of supportive psychotherapy.

Documentation needs to *follow* discussion with the patient. This includes not only documentation of short-term goals (for example, restoration of self-care behavior) but also considerations bearing on intermediate-term outcomes (for example, education in self-observation for early detection and reporting of symptoms consistent with relapse) and on long-term outcomes (for example, increased insight leading to a greater degree of autonomous function under conditions of stress). Where there are trade-offs among goals, those trade-offs need to be acknowledged.

Where treatment options are limited by economic or administrative considerations, the patient must be informed of this in as supportive a manner as possible as soon as is clinically feasible.

Where the initial managed care review denies benefits, patients should be supported in the appeals process.

Where the appeals process appears to be unfair, patients should be supported in obtaining their own consultations for second opinions from clinicians not directly affiliated with the treating institution.

Where such a consultation supports the treatment program agreed to by the clinician and the patient, and where benefits exist but have been denied by the managed care organization, such an external consultation can be the last resort before court. When the managed care organization refuses to recognize such an external consultation, there are a variety of legal options that the patient and family can exercise.

The importance of the treating clinician's exploring with the patient how to make best use of available resources is thus both clinical and administrative. Patient autonomy can be supported as clinicians and patients learn how to survive and even "surf" the great wave of managed care, which still seems to be on the rise. While the ethical and legal foundations for managing managed care are far from developed (Appelbaum, 1993; Wolf, 1994; Bursztajn, Feinbloom, Hamm, and Brodsky, 1990), this chapter's axiom and eight corollaries can be a rudimentary road map for clinicians working with patients hospitalized for psychiatric disorders.

Informed Consent

When we approach informed consent as a form to be signed by the patient in order to meet legal requirements, both the clinician and patient experience it as little more than a manipulation: clinical utility is absent and the legal value is dubious. On the other hand, when we understand that the criteria for informed consent derive meaning from a two-person process, the criteria can help build the doctor-patient alliance.

Quality care and the informed consent process are the wheel and axle of the vehicle of psychiatric inpatient diagnosis and treatment. The inpatient psychiatrist is legally mandated to obtain and document informed consent before administering all diagnostic and treatment interventions. In order to ensure that consent is *informed,* reasonable and appropriate information must be conveyed to the patient. The current standard for what kind of information and how much information the physician should disclose is that the physician should disclose all information that a reasonable person might want in deciding to accept or reject treatment: what the treatment consists of and the benefits and risks, alternative treatments and their benefits and risks, and no treatment and its benefits and risks. Since an exhaustive list of risks and alternatives is by no means practical or even possible in all cases, the clinician may wish to use a modified decision analytic sliding scale approach in determining how to engage the patient in the informed consent process. Stated simply, the greater the probability of an outcome or the greater the magnitude of the gain or loss associated with the outcome, the more incumbent it is upon the physician to enter that outcome into the dialogue.

The doctrine of informed consent stipulates that the patient must consent to a procedure before it is performed and that this consent be predicated on voluntary acceptance and competence in understanding reasonable information about the procedure or treatment. Failure to obtain patient consent may legally constitute battery; failure to meet the criteria for informed consent may constitute negligence. We can satisfy the criteria for informed consent by determining the patient's *voluntariness* of consent and *capacity* to take part in the informed consent procedure.

A patient's signed consent form is not considered evidence of voluntariness or competence. Thus, it is not a substitute for either the exploration I recommend or for documentation that such exploration took place. Its major use is as a reminder that exploration and documentation are necessary. When consent forms are routinely substituted for exploration and documentation, both quality of care and risk management suffer.

Voluntariness. In relation to informed consent, voluntariness means, most simply, that the patient made a choice in the absence of coercion. Some would argue that institutionalized individuals cannot voluntarily choose since their present needs and future wishes are tied to their caretakers' recommendations. Acceptance of this premise would deny institutionalized individuals the right to make any important decisions and seriously compromise the promotion of individual autonomy that informed consent seeks to achieve. Therefore, voluntariness of consent should be understood as free patient choice in the absence of coercion or undue influence. This applies equally to voluntarily or involuntarily hospitalized patients.

Capacity (competence). "The ability to understand rationally"—competence, in other words—is a legal concept determined by the court *(Kalmowitz v. Michigan Department of Mental Health).* Competence most often refers to the capacity to understand the nature and consequences of one's actions or decisions. Some individuals are recognized as generally incompetent, others as showing specific incompetence. In the latter group, the individual may be competent to arrive at personal decisions but not treatment decisions. The general rule today is that involuntary commitment does not presume incompetence. In fact, a committed mentally ill person is presumed competent unless legally adjudicated otherwise.

It is neither possible (because of limited resources) nor desirable to legally determine competence for each patient before the delivery of clinical services. The process of deciding to obtain a judicial competence evaluation is, therefore, integrated into the work of the inpatient unit. Psychiatrists and the courts use several tests for determining competency to consent to treatment. Certain populations appear at risk for incompetency: acutely psychotic patients who might exhibit delirium; chronic (long-term) institutionalized patients, who may have lost critical reasoning capacity; organically impaired patients; elderly senile patients; depressed patients, who may be generally hopeless about the future; and retarded patients (Gutheil, 1982). Psychiatrists should assess these groups if competency to consent to treatment is at all in question. To be judged psychologically competent, individuals should show an awareness of their current situation (living circumstances, relationships, health status, and so forth); possess a factual understanding of the issues, that is, exhibit a clear and realistic comprehension of the facts that bear upon decision making; and show the capacity to manipulate data rationally for decision making. These criteria can be applied to both general and specific competency assessments.

A primary concern to psychiatrists regarding competence of patients in an inpatient setting is consent to or refusal of treatment. Since precise competency standards for the treatment decision do not exist, psychiatrists should examine questionably incompetent patients and document findings. One approach is to use a consent form that has a written information component and an oral dialogue questions component to assess the level of the patient's understanding of information.

Patients who have already been judged by a court to be incompetent cannot then give informed consent. A court-appointed monitor or substitute decision maker must be obtained.

Special Situations

The requirements of informed consent do not apply to all situations. Emergencies, therapeutic privilege, waivers, and incompetency involve special legal and clinical consideration.

Emergencies. In medical emergencies, physicians may render medical services in the absence of formal consent if taking the time to secure consent (from the patient or substitute consenting adult) would pose a life-threatening delay in needed treatment. In psychiatry, treatment may be given in the absence of consent when patients become violent or self-mutilating and require intervention to prevent immediate harm to themselves or others. Unfortunately, the law to date does not generally recognize a broader sense of emergency, one that would include depressed patients in severe distress or even psychotic patients in overwhelming psychological pain (if they are nonviolent or not actively suicidal).

Therapeutic privilege. Another exception to informed consent standards is therapeutic privilege. If information about the patient's condition and treatment might be directly damaging to the patient, it can be withheld. However, such information cannot be withheld if the damage would be mediated solely by the decision of an adequately informed patient to refuse treatment. For example, the clinician's concern that a psychotic patient may refuse neuroleptics when informed of the risk of tardive dyskinesia is not sufficient grounds for withholding that information. In such a case, where the damage of a continuing untreated psychotic state is at issue, a careful competency assessment needs to be undertaken rather than invoking therapeutic privilege.

Waiver. The right of informed consent can be waived by the patient. The patient may say, "Tell me what to do. I don't want to know." This waiver should be respectfully explored by the clinician in order to assess the meaning of the patient's wish not to know, which may involve a degree of denial ranging from the healthy to the psychotic. Only such an exploration will suffice to document the patient's competence to waive informed consent. Blind compliance, as much as blind refusal, should alert the physician to potential pathology that may need to be addressed in the course of inpatient treatment.

In approaching informed consent as a two-person process, as described here, we seek to turn legal constraint to clinical advantage through the clinical dialogue. In doing so, the therapeutic alliance can be strengthened to withstand the uncertainty that characterizes inpatient treatment of high-risk populations.

Malpractice

Malpractice law is a subcategory of tort law, that branch of civil law concerned with providing redress for damages suffered as a consequence of a breach of duty. Malpractice is negligent or substandard practice by a professional or a failure to perform a duty that results in an injury to patient or client. Psychiatrists are liable for malpractice, though claims against psychiatrists are fewer than those against other medical specialties. The action taken in a tort is a demand for compensation for damages to the injured party. Four conditions must be met to have a malpractice claim.

Duty to care. In order for patients to allege that a physician's negligence caused them damage, they must first prove that the physician assumed a "duty to care," or a treatment relationship with them. Duty to care can be terminated if the patient is medically discharged or transferred to another facility or physician.

Negligence. The physician who takes on the duty to care for a specific patient also takes on the duty to care in a nonnegligent manner. Level of care is generally assessed against what other members of the medical specialty (with similar training and therapeutic orientation) would customarily do in a similar situation, that is, community standards (Gutheil, Bursztajn, Hamm, and Brodsky, 1983; Bursztajn, Gutheil, Hamm, and Brodsky, 1983). In some jurisdictions, however, the care given has been assessed as negligent in comparison with what a hypothetical "reasonable and prudent" practitioner might do or against an even more abstract risk-benefit standard for care. The prevailing current standard is the nationally recognized standard for psychiatric care. In practice, this is translated by courts to mean that the negligent practitioner or institution "deviated from accepted medical practice expected of a psychiatrist (or institution) in these circumstances." The existence of this standard derives in part from the presence of national journals, meetings, and organizations.

Harm. A physician is liable for damages only in the event that the breach of duty to care directly caused harm of a physical and/or emotional nature.

Causation. A physician who has established the duty to care for a patient in a nonnegligent way and has breached this duty is liable only if the alleged harm can be found to have been the direct consequence of this breach or the "proximate" result of the breach.

In summary, any patient suing a physician for malpractice must prove these four elements just described to be true by a preponderance of the evidence.

In recent years, one of the most frequent cause for action alleged in malpractice suits against psychiatrists has been psychiatric negligence leading to patient suicide. Other areas of litigation include medication side effects, improper diagnosis, the duty to inform, and sexual misconduct. I will review each of these briefly.

Suicide. The evidence demonstrates that patient suicide poses the second greatest number of malpractice claims against psychiatrists, accounting for more than 17 percent of all malpractice suits. The percentage increases when we include injury from a suicide attempt (American Psychiatric Association, 1990).

When the risk of suicide is present, as in the chronically suicidal borderline patient, the benefits of less restrictive care (for example, unlocked units or outpatient care) need to be weighed against the risks of being unable to prevent acting out of acute exacerbations of suicidal impulses (overdosing for example). In such cases, it is useful to engage the patients themselves—and where appropriate, their families—in the informed consent process. Planned transitions to less restrictive environments and leaves of absence provide an opportunity to assess and enhance a patient's capacity for engaging in dialogue and sharing responsibility—a capacity at the heart of therapeutic alliance building and the maturation process.

For inpatients, documentation of the clinical evaluation and decision to discharge is one protection against suit for the suicide of a recently discharged inpatient. When the patient is being discharged against medical advice, and the risk of suicide is thought to be chronic but the patient is not deemed committable, this reasoning should be shared with the patient and, when possible, the family. Documentation of the decision-making process, the consultation obtained, and the participation of patient and family is critical.

Inpatients thought to be at high risk of suicide constitute another medicolegal problem. Hospital procedures (be they close observation, one-to-one supervision, or some other intervention) should be openly reviewed. Although suicide proofing an inpatient unit remains a concept more platonic than realistic, the inpatient environment itself should be as free as possible of obvious opportunities for suicide, including, for example, insecure windows or access to sharp objects. A shared understanding by staff, patient, and family about what is being done and why in the context of an overall treatment plan is the best protection (Perr, 1985; Bursztajn, Gutheil, Brodsky, and Swagerty, 1988; Apter, Plutchik, and Sevy, 1989; Maltsburger, 1986).

Suicide litigation involves two main issues: first, whether the psychiatrist should have predicted that a patient was likely to commit self-harm, and second, if the risk was apparent, whether the psychiatrist took adequate precautions to protect the patient from self-harm. If a psychiatrist did not conclude that a hospitalized patient was in danger of self-harm and therefore did not take adequate precautions, the court will ask whether a reasonable and prudent psychiatrist would have predicted the risk. Courts do acknowledge the uncertainty of prediction in this area and will usually not hold a physician liable who exercised reasonable care. When the risk was apparent but the psychiatrist did not prevent the suicide, the courts question the adequacy of precautionary measures taken.

Medication Side Effects. Informed consent as an ongoing process (Gutheil, Bursztajn, and Brodsky, 1984) is particularly critical in an area as anxiety provoking to patients as medication side effects. And here, too, the process of informed consent allows the clinician the opportunity to turn legal constraints into clinical advantage (Wulsin, Bursztajn, and Gutheil, 1983). I shall focus on how to apply the process of informed consent to prescribing antipsychotic medication and informing the patient of the possible side effect of tardive dyskinesia. However, the following discussion applies to any medication with potentially serious side effects (for example, antidepressants and cardiac toxicity, antianxiety agents and addiction, lithium and renal toxicity).

Tardive dyskinesia (movement disorders of the face, tongue, and extremity muscles) is now an established side effect of antipsychotic medication. The development of tardive dyskinesia (TD) does not reflect negligence in administering antipsychotic drugs, for it can occur under optimal neuroleptic drug regimes. However, failure to warn patients of the risk of TD (as of any major side effect likely to occur) has in the recent past led to huge out-of-court settlements and in-court awards (Gelenberg, 1980; Appelbaum, Schaffner, and Meisel, 1985). Therefore, clinical care and malpractice liability concerns insist that psychiatrists fully inform patients of this side effect, obviously in an unthreatening and supportive fashion. Some researchers (recognizing the potential for malpractice suits in this area) suggest that written rather than oral informed consent be used with patients at high risk for TD (Davis, Schyre, and Parkovic, 1983). However, progress notes that document an ongoing process of review may be more clinically sound and no less a safeguard against suit.

Consent and liability issues with neuroleptics are of major import (American Psychiatric Association, 1979). The timing of consent is critical. If a patient is, by reason of psychosis, acutely incompetent and in need of emergency treatment, treat the patient and attempt to convey the relevant information; if treatment results in a restoration of competency, informed consent should await recompensation and should then be definitively obtained if and when further neuroleptic treatment is indicated (Muentz, 1985).

General counsel for the American Psychiatric Association (1979) urges reobtaining informed consent every six months for those patients on high doses of antipsychotic drugs. Only in an emergency should these drugs be used without consent. Therapeutic privilege, which holds that informed consent can be withheld if the physician believes that knowledge of risks would be directly detrimental to the patient, is another exception. However, most courts accept only extremely narrow instances of therapeutic privilege. As a rule, substitute consent from a legal guardian should be obtained instead of using therapeutic privilege.

An example of a case in this area is *Faigenbaum* v. *Cohen,* which involved the failure to warn about and diagnose tardive dyskinesia. In this case, TD was misdiagnosed as Huntington's chorea. The plaintiff sued the hospitals, drug companies, and physicians. The original verdict awarded $1.5 million to the plaintiff. (A current appeal is based on the state's claim of immunity from suit for its hospitals and physicians. The drug companies and private practice physicians have already settled.) In another case, *Hedin* v. *U.S.*, the court awarded $2.1 million to a veteran and an additional amount to his wife (for loss of companionship) on the basis of negligent prescription of neuroleptics by Veterans Administration physicians. The message to inpatient psychiatrists should be clear: always obtain informed consent before nonemergency treatment with neuroleptics.

As newer antipsychotic agents are developed and approved for clinical use and as their side effect profile may involve a lower risk of TD and a higher risk of other potentially irreversible serious side effects, the clinician will be responsible for reviewing the options and weighing their risks and benefits for the chronically ill patient. Where ongoing family treatment is part of the therapeutic approach to the chronically ill patient, the informed consent process can be extended to include the family. A psychiatrist in the often ambiguous role of medical backup to a nonmedical therapist should insist on meeting with the patient on an ongoing basis and be actively involved in educating both the patient and the nonmedical therapist about treatment options (Vasile and Gutheil, 1979; Bursztajn, Feinbloom, Hamm, and Brodsky, 1990). Blind prescribing carries with it not only the risks of negligent clinical care but also leaves open the possibility that the informed consent process will be aborted, leaving the clinician open to liability for negligently administering medication.

The initial use of high dosages of a high-potency neuroleptic and the failure to attempt to gradually wean the patient from such high dosages after a crisis represent a special kind of care and risk management problem. For example, *Leal* v. *Simon* resulted in a jury award of $2 million for the patient's pain and suffering as a result of the excessive use of haloperidol and $500,000 for care and maintenance services. In this case, the appellate courts acted to reduce jury awards; however, it is not unusual for damages to be assessed in excess of $1 million.

Improper Diagnosis. This category deserves explanation, for we are all aware that clinical diagnostic errors and ambiguities are inevitable. However, malpractice involving improper diagnosis does not pertain to human error in judgment. Rather, it applies to negligence, as in failing to use the diagnostic procedures and equipment that a prudent, competent psychiatrist would use to reach a diagnosis. An example of diagnostic negligence would be treating as a psychiatric disorder an organic disorder that should have been suspected and failing to obtain an internal medicine consultation.

Homicide and the Problem of Confidentiality. Although legal cases involving psychiatric patients who commit a violent act against a third party do not occur frequently, they may result in large financial awards. The parallel to suicide cases is apparent: both involve the uncertainty that surrounds the prediction of violence. Furthermore, instances of violence raise questions about whether and how the psychiatrist took prophylactic measures to prevent a potentially violent patient from causing harm. Courts have been less sympathetic towards psychiatrists' difficulties in predicting dangerousness towards others than they have been in cases involving violence toward the self (suicide).

A number of cases involve identifiable victims and the duty to protect (or to warn). These cases involve both outpatients and recently released inpatients. The outcome of most of these cases has held the psychiatrist liable for injuries to the victim when, first, the psychiatrist knew or should have known that the patient was likely to harm a specific individual, and second, the psychiatrist failed to warn or otherwise protect that individual. An often-quoted and, by now, famous case that held a therapist liable for failing to prevent a violent act towards a patient's victim was *Tarasoff* v. *Regents of the University of California.* In this instance, a former student contacted a school psychologist for therapy. The psychologist tried to initiate civil commitment of the young man based on the supposition that this patient might harm his ex-girlfriend, Tatiana Tarasoff. The university police who subsequently interviewed the young man decided on their own that he should not be committed. He murdered Tatiana Tarasoff several months thereafter. The family sued the university and the involved clinicians on the basis that they should have done more to protect the young woman. The California Supreme Court held that once a therapist does in fact determine, or under applicable professional standards reasonably should have determined, that a patient poses a serious danger of violence to others, the therapist bears a duty to exercise reasonable care to protect the foreseeable victim of that danger. The duty to protect (or warn) exists in many states when specific threats are made against specific victims. Some states go even further than the Tarasoff decision, holding that psychiatrists may be liable even if their patients harm persons not specified in advance (Appelbaum, 1984).

While the courts have often found the clinician liable in cases in which (in hindsight) the violation of confidentiality would have resulted in saving the life of a third party, an opposing trend is also noted. Recently both Massachusetts and New Hampshire courts indicated that in nonemergency cases, the clinician may be found liable for breaking confidentiality (*Commonwealth of Massachusetts* v. *Cokrin*)! In view of these opposing trends, clinicians can avoid court-created paralysis by carefully documenting their reasoning and, when in doubt, seeking consultation.

A number of states, Massachusetts among them, have attempted to avoid court-induced paralysis with legislation that clearly spells out a therapist's duties and therapeutic options for discharging such duties. While such legislation is often initiated by state psychiatric societies in conjunction with other disciplinary societies and highly touted as a panacea for judicial intrusion into the treatment domain, it remains to be proven whether the substitution of legislative for judicial limitation of clinical autonomy and treatment options in high-risk cases truly decreases the risk of liability following a tragic outcome.

Sexual Misconduct and Other Boundary Violations. The intensity of affect and the states of regression of many patients often favor various boundary violations. These include inappropriate socialization and fraternization, exchanges of gifts and money, special favors, and the entire spectrum of sexual misconduct. While most of these are problems of therapy and administration, the last has an additional weight.

While charges of sexual misconduct have been brought against physicians in various specialties, a psychiatrist who engages in sexual contact with a patient is clearly betraying the patient's trust. The rule clearly stated by the

American Psychiatric Association code of ethics is that any sexual activity between patient and therapist represents improper behavior on the therapist's part (Gutheil and Appelbaum, 1982). More recently, the breach of ethics has been extended to cover sexual relations with former patients. In addition, both civil and criminal prosecution for battery may be charged when such misconduct, however rationalized, occurs. It should be noted that the current malpractice insurance policy offered to APA members specifically excludes coverage for liability incurred on the basis of sexual misconduct.

Inpatient clinicians should be particularly sensitive to the vulnerability of hospitalized patients and staff to respond to feelings of frustration, hopelessness, and helplessness by a flight toward sexualization. Clinicians should be aware that under the doctrine of *respondeat superior* (the vicarious responsibility of superiors), they may be held liable for sexual acting out with patients by staff members under their direct supervision. The doctrine of *respondeat superior* continues to enlarge in scope. Where sexual acting out has occurred by treatment team staff, the treating clinician, clinical administrator, and host institution may all be considered negligent. Where the early cases of negligence involved the failure to prevent such sexual contact once it came to light, the most recent trend clearly points to a finding of negligence irrespective of professed ignorance on the part of the supervising clinician or institution. Failure to provide an educational program and ongoing clinical supervision regarding the ethical issues and countertransference feelings raised in the course of treating seriously ill (and often previously abused) patients and failing to probe credentials thoroughly is well below accepted standards for supervision (Bursztajn, 1990).

Inpatient units treating populations at high risk for sexual exploitation (for example, adolescents or substance abusers) can meet the standard of care only if they provide adequate psychiatric supervision of clinical staff. Staff should be supported in understanding sexually provocative patient behavior and their own fantasies and feelings as transference and countertransference reactions to be clinically addressed.

Other situations that may invoke the potential for malpractice suits include the patient's right to sign him- or herself out of treatment, refusal of specific treatments, seclusion and restraint, and involuntary discharge.

Conclusion

While delivery of quality care, documentation, consultation, and familiarity with your state's restrictions are critical avenues of malpractice prevention, they are not the limits of preventive approaches. Physician sharing of the uncertainty of diagnosis, treatment, and outcome with patients is yet another malpractice prevention strategy (Gutheil, Bursztajn, and Brodsky, 1984). Malpractice suits in medicine often result from patient and family disappointment and helplessness in the face of tragic outcomes, rather than negligence. Informed consent, when practiced pro forma, often carries the suggestion of a guarantee and leads to unrealistic hopes. Instead, I recommend that informed consent be used as a starting point in establishing a true therapeutic alliance. Uncertainty is then mutually acknowledged and clinical decision making becomes a dialogue that is characteristic of the psychiatrist-patient relationship at its best. It is imperative to bear in mind that a clinical alliance rather than a legal adversary process is the goal of treatment.

References

American Psychiatric Association. *Tardive Dyskinesia: Report of the American Psychiatric Association Task Force on Late Neurological Effects of Antipsychotic Drugs.* Task Force Report no. 18. Washington, D.C., American Psychiatric Association, 1979.

American Psychiatric Association. Data supplied by the insurers of APA members, 1990.

Appelbaum, P. S. "The Expansion of Liability for Patients' Violent Acts." *Hospital & Community Psychiatry,* 1984, *35,* 13–14.

Appelbaum, P. S. "Legal Liability and Managed Care." *American Psychologist,* March 1993, pp. 251–257.

Appelbaum, P. S., Schaffner, K., and Meisel, A. "Responsibility and Compensation for Tardive Dyskinesia." *American Journal of Psychiatry,* 1985, *142,* 806–810.

Apter, A., Plutchik, R., and Sevy, S. "Defense Mechanisms in Risk of Suicide and Risk of Violence." *American Journal of Psychiatry,* 1989, *146,* 1027–1031.

Bursztajn, H. J. "Supervisory Responsibility for Prevention of Supervisee-Patient Sexual Contact." Paper presented at the Massachusetts Psychiatric Society, Newton, Mass., Mar. 10, 1990.

Bursztajn, H. J., Feinbloom, R. I., Hamm, R. M., and Brodsky, A. *Medical Choices, Medical Chances: How Patients, Families, and Physicians Can Cope with Uncertainty.* New York: Routledge, Chapman & Hall, 1990.

Bursztajn, H. J., Gutheil, T. G., Brodsky, A., and Swagerty, E. "Magical Thinking, Suicide, and Malpractice Litigation." *Bulletin of the American Academy of Psychiatry and the Law,* 1988, *16,* 369–377.

Bursztajn, H., Gutheil, T. G., Hamm, R. M., and Brodsky, A. "Subjective Data and Suicide Assessment in the Light of Recent Legal Developments. Part II: Clinical Uses of Legal Standards in the Interpretation of Subjective Data." *International Journal of Law and Psychiatry,* 1983, *6,* 331–350.

Commonwealth of Massachusetts v. *Cokrin,* SJC-3671 (1985); 493 A2D 472 (Apr. 18, 1985 S.Ct. NH).

Davis, J. M., Schyre, P. M., and Parkovic, I. "Clinical and Legal Issues in Neuroleptic Use." *Clinical Neuropharmacology,* 1983, *6,* 117–128.

Faigenbaum v. *Cohen.* Reported in *Clinical Psychiatry News,* 1985, *5,* 31.

Gelenberg, A. "375,000 for Tardive Dyskinesia." *Biological Therapies in Psychiatry,* 1980, *3,* 41–42.

Gutheil, T. G., and Appelbaum, P. S. *Clinical Handbook of Psychiatry and the Law.* New York: McGraw-Hill, 1982.

Gutheil, T. G., Bursztajn, H. J., and Brodsky, A. "Malpractice Prevention Through the Sharing of Uncertainty: Informed Consent and the Therapeutic Alliance." *New England Journal of Medicine,* 1984, *311,* 49–51.

Gutheil, T. G., Bursztajn, H. J., Hamm, R. M., and Brodsky, A. "Subjective Data and Suicide Assessment in the Light of Recent Legal Developments. Part 1: Malpractice Prevention and the Use of Subjective Data." *International Journal of Law and Psychiatry,* 1983, *6,* 317–329.

Hedin v. *U.S.* Reported in *Clinical Psychiatry News,* 1985, *5,* 31. *Kalmowitz* v. *Michigan Department of Mental Health,* Div. No. 73–19434 AW, Circuit Court of Wayne Cty, Mich., 1973, 13 Criminal L Rep 2452.

Leal v. *Simon*, 542 N.Y.S. 2d 328 (1989).
Maltsburger, J. T. *Suicide Risk: The Formulation of Clinical Judgment.* New York: New York University Press, 1986.
Muentz, M. R. "Overcoming Resistance to Talking to Patients About Tardive Dyskinesia." *Hospital & Community Psychiatry*, 1985, *36*, 283–287.
Perr, I. N. "Psychiatric Malpractice Issues." In S. Rachlin (ed.), *Legal Encroachment on Psychiatric Practice.* San Francisco, Jossey-Bass, 1985.
Tarasoff v. *Regents of the University of California,* 131 Cal Reptr 14 (Calif. 76).
Vasile, R. G., and Gutheil, T. G. "The Psychiatrist as Medical Backup: Ambiguity in the Delegation of Clinical Responsibility." *American Journal of Psychiatry*, 1979, *136*, 1292–1296.
Wolf, S. M. "Health Care Reform and the Future of Physician Ethics." *Hastings Center Report*, March–April 1994, pp. 28–41.
Wulsin, L. R., Bursztajn, H. J., and Gutheil, T. G. "Unexpected Clinical Features of the Tarasoff Decision: The Therapeutic Alliance and the Duty to Warn." *American Journal of Psychiatry*, 1983, *140*, 601–603.

HAROLD J. BURSZTAJN, M.D., is co-director of the Program in Psychiatry and the Law of the Harvard Medical School at the Massachusetts Mental Health Center.

INDEX

Ordering Information

New Directions for Mental Health Services is a series of paperback books that presents timely and readable volumes on subjects of concern to clinicians, administrators, and others involved in the care of the mentally disabled. Each volume is devoted to one topic and includes a broad range of authoritative articles written by noted specialists in the field. Books in the series are published quarterly in Spring, Summer, Fall, and Winter and are available for purchase by subscription as well as individually.

Subscriptions for 1994 cost $54.00 for individuals (a savings of 25 percent over single-copy prices) and $75.00 for institutions, agencies, and libraries. Please do not send institutional checks for personal subscriptions. Standing orders are accepted.

Single copies cost $17.95 when payment accompanies order. (California, New Jersey, New York, and Washington, D.C., residents please include appropriate sales tax.) All orders will be charged postage and handling.

Discounts for quantity orders are available. Please write to the address below for information.

All orders must include either the name of an individual or an official purchase order number. Please submit your order as follows:

Subscriptions: specify series and year subscription is to begin
Single copies: include individual title code (such as MHS59)

Mail all orders to:

Jossey-Bass Publishers
350 Sansome Street
San Francisco, California 94104-1342

For subscription sales outside of the United States, contact any international subscription agency or Jossey-Bass directly.

Other Titles Available in the
New Directions for Mental Health Services Series
H. Richard Lamb, Editor-in-Chief

MHS62 Family Interventions in Mental Illness, *Agnes B. Hatfield*
MHS61 Mental Health Care in Canada, *Leona L. Bachrach, Paula Goering, Donald Wasylenki*
MHS60 Innovations in Japanese Mental Health Services, *James M. Mandiberg*
MHS59 Managed Mental Health Care, *William Goldman, Saul Feldman*
MHS58 A Nursing Perspective on Severe Mental Illness, *Linda Chafetz*
MHS57 Medical-Surgical Psychiatry: Treating Psychiatric Aspects of Physical Disorders, *Troy L. Thompson II*
MHS56 Innovative Community Mental Health Programs, *Leonard I. Stein*
MHS55 Treating Diverse Disorders with Psychotherapy, *David Greenfeld*
MHS54 Neurobiological Disorders in Children and Adolescents, *Enid Peschel, Richard Peschel, Carol W. Howe, James W. Howe*
MHS53 Effective Psychiatric Rehabilitation, *Robert Paul Liberman*
MHS52 Psychiatric Outreach to the Mentally Ill, *Neal L. Cohen*
MHS51 Treating Victims of Child Sexual Abuse, *John Briere*
MHS50 Dual Diagnosis of Major Mental Illness and Substance Disorder, *Kenneth Minkoff, Robert Drake*
MHS49 Administrative Issues in Public Mental Health, *Stuart L. Keill*
MHS48 Psychiatric Aspects of AIDS and HIV Infection, *Stephen M. Goldfinger*
MHS47 Treating Personality Disorders, *David A. Adler*
MHS46 Using Psychodynamic Principles in Public Mental Health, *Terry A. Kupers*
MHS45 New Developments in Psychiatric Rehabilitation, *Arthur T. Meyerson, Phyllis Solomon*
MHS43 Paying for Services: Promises and Pitfalls of Capitation, *David Mechanic, Linda H. Aiken*
MHS41 Legal Implications of Hospital Policies and Practices, *Robert D. Miller*
MHS40 Clinical Case Management, *Maxine Harris, Leona L. Bachrach*
MHS39 Serving the Chronically Mentally Ill in an Urban Setting: The Massachusetts Mental Health Center Experience, *Miles F. Shore, Jon E. Gudeman*
MHS38 Differing Approaches to Partial Hospitalization, *Kenneth Goldberg*
MHS36 Improving Mental Health Services: What the Social Sciences Can Tell Us, *David Mechanic*
MHS35 Leona Bachrach Speaks: Selected Speeches and Lectures, *Leona L. Bachrach*
MHS34 Families of the Mentally Ill: Meeting the Challenges, *Agnes B. Hatfield*
MHS32 Treating Anxiety Disorders, *Rodrigo A. Muñoz*
MHS31 Eating Disorders, *Félix E. F. Larocca*
MHS29 The Elderly and Chronic Mental Illness, *Nancy S. Abramson, Jean K. Quam, Mona Wasow*
MHS22 Patterns of Adolescent Self-Image, *Daniel Offer, Eric Ostrov, Kenneth I. Howard*
MHS14 The Young Adult Chronic Patient, *Bert Pepper, Hilary Ryglewicz*